The GP Guide to Secondary Care

Radcliffe Medical Press

© 2000 Keith Hopcroft

Radcliffe Medical Press Ltd
18 Marcham Road, Abingdon, Oxon OX14 1AA

British Library Cataloguing in Publication Data

A catalogue record for this book is available from the British Library.

ISBN 1 85775 398 4

Typeset by Joshua Associates Ltd, Oxford
Indexed by Dr Laurence Errington
Printed and bound by TJ International Ltd, Padstow, Cornwall

CONTENTS

PREFACE

GPs have become accustomed to coping with an ever expanding role. However, hospital-based investigations remain – by definition – outside the primary care remit. This begs the following question: why a book for GPs on secondary care investigations? There are two main reasons.

First, the GP is still, for most patients, an accessible, trusted and reliable source of information. So when individuals under hospital follow-up find themselves dazed and confused by the hi-tech intentions of their specialists, it is to their GP that they turn. All family doctors will be familiar with such scenarios – consultants too rushed or cavalier to provide a full explanation, or patients too fearful to request or retain relevant information. As a result, it often falls to the GP to pick up the pieces of an out-patient appointment – for example, by explaining the purpose of an MRI scan, commenting on the limitations of an EEG or advising on just how painful electromyography might be. The problem is, of course, that rapid retrieval of basic facts about such tests has until now been virtually impossible.

Secondly, GPs have open access to an increasing and at times bewildering array of hospital-based investigations. X-rays and blood tests are, of course, old hat. However, depending on area, interest and policy, some GPs can now let their investigative imaginations run riot by arranging, for example, ultrasounds, Holter monitoring or MRI scans. Indeed, the germ of the idea that became this book was implanted in me on the day when I heard that I could refer patients for open-access echocardiography. On the one hand, I was delighted at the improved service I could offer. On the other, I was embarrassed to realise that I did not know who I should 'echo', what to warn them it would be like or how to interpret the results. Such naïvety is becoming less permissible. With greater access to secondary care investigations comes increasing responsibility to use them properly, especially in the context of clinical governance, primary care groups and financial constraints.

This book aims to plug these gaps in our knowledge. It provides a compendium of all those hospital-based tests to which we currently have – or will soon develop – access. It also includes the rather more specialised tests available only to the relevant consultant, but which we might end up having to explain to perplexed patients. If the book enables us to order secondary care investigations confidently and rationally, and to answer our patients' queries with authority, then it will have done its job.

Keith Hopcroft
January 2000

HOW TO USE THIS BOOK

The vast majority of GPs are perfectly comfortable with the appropriate use of basic X-rays and blood tests, and numerous books and guidelines exist to resolve any particular dilemmas. This book therefore focuses on the more complex, specialised or invasive hospital-based investigations that are of relevance to GPs.

The investigations themselves are arranged according to speciality. If a quick scan of the relevant chapter's contents does not reveal the test in question, then the index should oblige.

Each chapter is written by a specialist in the field, whose brief was to cover the most common investigations and to include others which might be less familiar but are relevant to GPs. Such a book cannot be completely exhaustive, so a balance has been struck by aiming for a reasonably comprehensive coverage while avoiding cluttering the pages with the overly esoteric.

To aid retrieval of information, most of the investigations are dealt with in a consistent manner, using the following headings.

- **DESCRIPTION:** a brief technical description of the investigation.
- **INDICATIONS:** the clinical situations in which the test is particularly useful.
- **POTENTIAL FINDINGS:** the interpretation of the results, including their relevance and implications.
- **RELATED INVESTIGATIONS:** the limitations of the test and a brief description of other tests which might be considered simultaneously, alternatively or subsequently.
- **PATIENT ADVICE:** a description of what the test is like for the patient, including pre-test preparation and post-test effects.
- **GP ADVICE:** a description of pre-test work-up, post-test adverse effects and how to manage them, and general considerations.

LIST OF CONTRIBUTORS

Peter Barnes, Professor of Respiratory Medicine, National Heart and Lung Institute, Imperial College of Science, Technology and Medicine, London

Ciaran Brady, Clinical Research Fellow, Department of Uro-Neurology, National Hospital for Neurology and Neurosurgery, London

Vin Diwaker, Specialist Registrar in Paediatrics, Birmingham Children's Hospital, Birmingham

Ian Fentiman, Professor of Surgical Oncology, Guy's Hospital, London

John Hampton, Professor of Cardiology, Department of Cardiovascular Medicine, University Hospital, Nottingham

Deirdre Kelly, Reader in Paediatric Hepatology, Birmingham Children's Hospital, Birmingham

Michael Laker, Reader and Consultant in Clinical Biochemistry and Metabolic Medicine/Medical Director, Newcastle upon Tyne Hospitals NHS Trust, Royal Victoria Infirmary, Newcastle upon Tyne

Hunter Maclean, Consultant Ophthalmic Surgeon, Queen Alexander Hospital, Portsmouth

Jeremy Nightingale, Consultant Gastroenterologist, Leicester Royal Infirmary, Leicester

Brian O'Reilly, Consultant ENT Surgeon, Basildon Hospital, Basildon

Elizabeth S Payne, Consultant Obstetrician and Gynaecologist, Princess of Wales Women's Unit, Birmingham Heartlands Hospital, Birmingham

Richard Rawlins, Consultant Orthopaedic Surgeon, Bedford Hospital, Bedford

David Reilly, Consultant General and Vascular Surgeon, Wirral Hospital NHS Trust, Arrowe Park Hospital, Wirral

Atul Sinha, Research Fellow in Gastroenterology, Leicester Royal Infirmary, Leicester

Robert Stirling, Clinical Research Fellow, National Heart and Lung Institute, Imperial College of Science, Technology and Medicine, London

Mark Temple, Consultant Nephrologist, Birmingham Heartlands Hospital, Birmingham

Henry G Watson, Consultant Haematologist, Department of Haematology, Aberdeen Royal Infirmary, Aberdeen

Stuart Wood, General Practitioner, Glasgow, and Senior Lecturer in General Practice, University of Glasgow

Carolyn A Young, Consultant Neurologist, The Watson Centre for Neurology and Neurosurgery, Fazakerley, Liverpool

ACKNOWLEDGEMENTS

I would like to thank several people who were particularly helpful in the production of this book.

- Heidi Allen and Paula Moran for their encouragement, patience and lunches.
- All of the contributors, who produced such high-quality material – even those who delighted in indulging in brinkmanship with the deadlines.
- Denise, Henry and William for reminding me that there is life beyond a VDU.
- Whoever succeeded in arranging open-access echocardiography in my locality, as this was the inspiration for the book.

BREAST

Mammography

Ultrasound

Magnetic resonance imaging (MRI)

Fine-needle aspiration cytology (FNAC)

Core-needle biopsy

Triple assessment

BREAST

Ian Fentiman

Most women with breast symptoms can safely be reassured after sympathetically taking a history, performing a thorough clinical examination and giving a clear explanation of the physiological rather than pathological cause.

Appropriate indications for referral to a breast clinic are the presence of a lump, localised nodularity, skin dimpling, unilateral nipple inversion or nipple/areola eczema.

Mammography

DESCRIPTION

Mammography consists of breast X-rays taken after compression of the tissue to obtain cranio-caudal and oblique views.

INDICATIONS

- Women with breast symptoms aged > 40 years.
- To determine the radiological appearance of the region of concern and to detect clinically impalpable abnormalities.
- In patients with cancer, mammography may help to establish the extent of the disease and to check for contralateral disease (which occurs synchronously in 5% of cases).
- The National Breast Screening Programme is open to all women aged 50 to 64 years, who are recalled every 3 years. Women aged over 65 years are eligible, but are not included in the call–recall system.

POTENTIAL FINDINGS

- Asymmetrical breast tissue density: this is often benign, but can result from a cancer.
- Single or multiple opacities: if well defined, a benign cause is likely. An irregular outline suggests malignancy or an inflammatory reaction.

- Distortion of breast tissue, sometimes of stellate appearance, resulting from fibrosis around small tumours or at the site of a previous surgical operation.
- Macrocalcification in fibrocystic disease, fibroadenomas and old suture material.
- Microcalcification which is fine and dispersed is usually benign.
- Microcalcification which is of irregular shape and size is likely to be the result of ductal carcinoma *in situ*. This may sometimes be associated with an opacity or stromal distortion in patients with invasive breast cancer.

RELATED INVESTIGATIONS

- Ultrasound to determine whether opacities are fluid-filled or solid.
- Compression/magnification view to determine the nature of fine microcalcification.
- Compression/magnification view of an area of dubious scarring or possible superimposition of benign areas.
- Stereotactic core-needle biopsy for establishing a tissue diagnosis of an impalpable lesion.

PATIENT ADVICE

- Mammography can be uncomfortable but is only rarely very painful.
- Pressure is required to obtain the best images.
- Most of the abnormalities that are detected are benign.
- Some cancers can be missed, and any subsequent breast lumps need to be assessed.

GP ADVICE

- Referral for mammography/ultrasound is a very high-risk strategy because patients with breast lumps or localised nodularity require triple assessment, namely clinical examination, imaging and a tissue diagnosis.
- Obtaining a normal ultrasound or mammogram in a patient with a lump is not sufficient evidence to dismiss the lesion as benign.

Ultrasound

DESCRIPTION

- Ultrasound is a technique that uses the reflection and refraction of ultrasonic wavelengths to produce images.
- Because there is no exposure to ionising radiation, the technique can be repeated as often as is necessary.
- Ultrasound should not be regarded as a form of breast screening in pre-menopausal women.

INDICATIONS

- The investigation of palpable lumps or mammographic opacities to determine whether they are solid or cystic.
- The measurement (sometimes) of the dimensions of a lesion.
- The assessment of the margins of a lesion such as a fibroadenoma to determine the definition of the margins.

POTENTIAL FINDINGS

- Confirmation that a lump has well-defined anterior and posterior walls with no internal echoes and that it is cystic, allowing either aspiration or reassurance alone.
- When the ultrasound examination shows a mass lesion with displacement of breast architecture and well-defined internal echoes and borders, it is likely that the lump is a fibroadenoma.
- Irregularity of margins, heterogeneous internal echoes and disruption of normal tissue planes are suggestive of malignancy.

RELATED INVESTIGATIONS

- Ultrasound-guided fine-needle aspiration or core-needle biopsy.
- Ultrasound guide-needle localisation prior to excision of impalpable lesions.

PATIENT ADVICE

- A painless test to distinguish between solid and fluid-filled abnormalities.
- Not a cancer screening test.

GP ADVICE

- Not a cancer screening test.
- Not for the evaluation of nodular regions within the breast.
- If ultrasound examination has shown a palpable lump to be cystic, aspiration by the GP is justified.

Magnetic resonance imaging (MRI)

DESCRIPTION

- The nuclei of elements such as hydrogen and phosphorus are magnetic, and when exposed to a pulse of high magnetic field they align in the direction of the field.
- When the pulse is switched off, the nuclei emit detectable radio-signals as they return to their prior configuration.

INDICATIONS

- Determination of the extent of malignancy within the affected and contra-lateral breast.
- Differentiation between scar tissue and local relapse in patients who have undergone breast conservation therapy.

POTENTIAL FINDINGS

- Mammography may underestimate the extent of both invasive and non-invasive breast cancer, and the true extent may be revealed by MRI.
- An area of suspicious recurrence may be shown to be malignant by demonstrating enhancement (increasing whiteness) after injection of gadolinium-diethylenetriamine pentacetic acid (Gd-DTPA).

RELATED INVESTIGATIONS

- Sometimes malignancy may be detectable only by MRI, and so very specialised needle-localisation biopsy is necessary using non-ferrous tungsten needles.
- Ultrasound is used when there is an MRI-detected lesion, as there may be a detectable change in density at the site of the lesion which may enable an easier localisation using the ultrasound probe.

PATIENT ADVICE

- MRI does not involve exposure to ionising radiation, but the machinery involved may intimidate those of a nervous predisposition.
- Patients who suffer from claustrophobia may be unable to tolerate the confined space and the noise involved in MRI scanning.
- All ferrous objects must be removed before the examination, and patients who have undergone prior surgery with insertion of metallic implants such as pacemakers cannot undergo MRI.

GP ADVICE

- Patients can be reassured that the test is painless and safe although it may seem very daunting.

Fine-needle aspiration cytology (FNAC)

DESCRIPTION

- This is the most widely used test for making a pre-operative diagnosis of breast cancer, in which a needle attached to an empty syringe is inserted into a suspicious lesion.
- The needle plunger is withdrawn to create a negative pressure, and the needle is then passed approximately 10 times through the lesion, changing the angle to obtain as wide a sample as possible.
- The needle is withdrawn and the contents are expelled on to a glass slide which is smeared on to a second slide.
- One slide is air-dried and the other is fixed in ethyl alcohol; both are stained.
- Washings into normal saline may also be sent for examination.

- These slides are examined by a pathologist with special training in cyto-pathology.

INDICATIONS

- To confirm that a suspected benign lesion is not malignant.
- To determine whether a suspected breast cancer contains malignant cells.
- To confirm that a suspicious node or skin nodule is malignant.

POTENTIAL FINDINGS

Cytology is reported on a 1–5 scale as follows:

- C1, acellular specimen (non-diagnostic);
- C2, benign epithelial cells present;
- C3, atypical but probably benign cells;
- C4, atypical and probably malignant cells;
- C5, malignant cells.

RELATED INVESTIGATIONS

- Many centres now carry out core-needle biopsy in addition to FNAC so that a histological diagnosis of invasive breast cancer can be made.
- Some cytologists will give a grade I/II/III for malignant cells.
- Both oestrogen and progesterone receptors can be determined in FNAC specimens.

PATIENT ADVICE

- There may be some discomfort associated with FNAC, but the procedure is relatively quick and will be carried out at the time of a visit to a one-stop clinic.
- If a breast lump is suspected to be a fibroadenoma and the patient does not wish to undergo surgery, both FNAC and ultrasound examination are necessary to confirm the nature of the lesion.
- *See also* comments under 'Triple assessment'.

GP ADVICE

- For a woman with a definite lump, a C1 result means that the test must be repeated or the lump removed.
- For a patient with an area of nodularity but no lump, a C1 result is acceptable.
- A C5 result means that malignancy is present, but it does not distinguish between invasive and non-invasive cancer.

Core-needle biopsy

DESCRIPTION

- A technique for obtaining a histological specimen from a lump which is presumed to be malignant.
- Core biopsy has a sensitivity of 80–90% – that is, it will make a pre-operative diagnosis in eight or nine out of every 10 cancers.

INDICATIONS

- Making a pre-operative diagnosis of breast cancer.
- In a young woman with a suspected fibroadenoma, core biopsy may be used to obtain a representative specimen if the patient wishes to avoid excision biopsy.

POTENTIAL FINDINGS

- Confirmation that a lump is an invasive carcinoma.
- Only non-invasive cancer is present, indicating the need for an excision biopsy.
- No malignancy is found in a suspicious lump, indicating the need for an excision biopsy.
- Confirmation that a discrete lump is a fibroadenoma.

RELATED INVESTIGATIONS

- Core biopsy may be combined with FNAC to maximise the likelihood of making a pre-operative diagnosis in a patient with suspected breast cancer.
- Negative core biopsy should not be taken as proof that a lump is benign, and so excision biopsy is necessary.

- Core biopsy may be used after stereotactic localisation to determine the nature of a mammographically detected lesion.

PATIENT ADVICE

- Core-needle biopsy is carried out after injection of local anaesthetic.
- It is rarely painful.
- The main complication after the procedure is bruising.
- *See also* comments under 'Triple assessment'.

GP ADVICE

- Successful core biopsy can significantly reduce the number of diagnostic excision biopsies. This results in an out-patient diagnosis of breast cancer.
- In patients with large primary tumours, core biopsy can not only make the diagnosis but also determine the hormone-receptor status of the tumour. This enables first-line endocrine therapy in appropriate cases to shrink the tumour pre-operatively and allow breast conservation therapy.
- In some patients, core biopsy may be used prior to cytotoxic chemotherapy as first-line treatment.

Triple assessment

DESCRIPTION

- Patients with breast lumps or localised nodularity require triple assessment, namely clinical examination, imaging and a tissue diagnosis. After clinical assessment, mammography and often ultrasound examination will be performed, following which a core biopsy or FNAC will be carried out.

INDICATIONS

- Women with suspected breast cancers who are seen urgently in one-stop clinics.
- Young women with suspected fibroadenomas, because this diagnosis cannot be made on clinical grounds alone.

POTENTIAL FINDINGS

- Confirmation that a lump is benign.
- Confirmation of malignancy.
- An equivocal result, so that a diagnostic biopsy is recommended.

RELATED INVESTIGATIONS

- Despite a benign diagnosis, some patients will still wish to undergo excision biopsy or an incision biopsy from a large area of nodularity.

PATIENT ADVICE

- For those with cancer, the diagnosis may be given either at the one-stop clinic or a few days later in a results clinic, and the patient should be encouraged to attend with a relative or friend.

GP ADVICE

- Only 1 in 10 symptomatic patients referred to hospital will be found to have malignancy.

CARDIOLOGY

Echocardiography

Exercise testing

Ambulatory ECG recording

Cardiac catheterisation

Ambulatory blood pressure recording

Radionuclide investigations

Magnetic resonance imaging (MRI)

CARDIOLOGY

John Hampton

Hospital cardiologists and cardiovascular physicians have at their disposal a range of techniques for investigation of cardiovascular functions. These are increasingly being made available to GPs by direct access, but certain principles apply to all of them.

- A patient's history remains the most important pointer to diagnosis.

- The physical examination is especially valuable in cardiovascular disease, and it is essential not to allow an over-dependence on an apparently sophisticated investigation to supplant the skills of clinical examination.

- Some investigations are inherently costly, either because of the capital costs of the equipment or because of the salary cost of technicians. Many hospitals are inadequately equipped for their own needs and may have to ration or refuse direct access to investigations on pragmatic grounds.

- Most cardiological investigations require interpretation, and an interpretation is to some extent an opinion. There is little point in direct access to an investigation which leads to an incomprehensible clinical report. Although a hospital physician may be able to interpret the technicalities, his or her comments may not be helpful if he or she has not seen the patient.

- Direct access is not appropriate for investigations that involve a risk – for example, cardiac catheterisation – where the clinician who is to take responsibility must see the patient beforehand.

Echocardiography

DESCRIPTION

Echocardiography involves taking a moving picture of the heart by reflected ultrasound. The technique produces pictures which represent 'slices' of the heart, and interpreting these pictures requires skill and experience. GPs are unlikely ever to see enough echocardiograms to be able to interpret the recordings for themselves, and so have to rely on technical reports. Technicians' reports include a large number of measurements, the significance of which the GP will find difficult to interpret. Most GPs find some form of clinical comment by a cardiologist essential.

INDICATIONS

The main uses of echocardiography are as follows:

- to establish the cause of heart failure in a patient for whom the diagnosis is in no doubt;
- to show whether there are structural abnormalities in the heart which might be responsible for heart failure, thereby providing circumstantial evidence that a patient's symptoms are due to heart failure;
- to help to investigate breathlessness;
- to assess the significance of heart murmurs;
- to screen healthy subjects who have a family history of cardiomyopathy, especially hypertrophic cardiomyopathy.

POTENTIAL FINDINGS

- The technical report may say that it was difficult to obtain clear pictures. This usually indicates obesity or chronic lung disease.
- Valves may be described as normal or thickened. Valve stenosis – especially aortic stenosis – will be quantified by an estimate of the pressure drop across the valve. An aortic valve 'gradient' of less than 40 mmHg indicates mild stenosis, a gradient of 40–70 mmHg is moderate and a gradient greater than 70 mmHg indicates severe stenosis that probably needs surgery.
- A minor degree of mitral regurgitation is almost universal, and is of no significance.
- A dilated left ventricle and/or a description of poor contraction suggests that heart failure is, or will become, a problem, and provides an indication for the use of angiotensin-converting enzyme (ACE) inhibitors. The 'ejection fraction' (the proportion of blood expelled from the heart with each beat) can be derived from the echo, but the measurement is not reliable. It should be greater than 50%, but even a low ejection fraction does not necessarily mean that a patient has heart failure. It simply means that there is cardiac malfunction, and that heart failure is possible.

Any structural abnormality, including valve disease, a dilated left ventricle or a dilated left atrium, indicates the need for anticoagulants in a patient with atrial fibrillation.

RELATED INVESTIGATIONS

- A patient with a completely normal electrocardiogram (ECG) is unlikely to have an abnormal echocardiogram, although this is not an absolute rule.

- The echocardiogram provides a better assessment of heart size than a chest X-ray. The main value of the chest X-ray is in assessing the presence of pulmonary congestion.

PATIENT ADVICE

- No preparation is necessary.

- A patient must expect to undress to the waist.

- The test will take about 20 minutes; it will be performed in a darkened room and the moving heart can be seen on a television screen.

- The recorder may produce some loud noises which are not actually made by the heart, but which are an artificial representation of flowing blood.

GP ADVICE

- The more information the GP provides on a request card, and the more clearly the problem is described, the more valuable the report will be. A hospital department should not accept a request with an inadequate description of the patient's symptoms and signs.

- If a patient has symptoms that might be due to cardiac disease (breathlessness, ankle swelling, syncope) then the presence of an echocardiographic abnormality probably gives an indication of the cause of the symptom. For example, a patient who is breathless and has impaired left ventricular function on echo probably has heart failure (but could, alternatively, have either chest disease or anaemia) and will probably benefit from ACE inhibitor therapy.

Exercise testing

DESCRIPTION

Exercise testing can be performed on a static bicycle or, more often, on a treadmill. On the treadmill the 'Bruce protocol' is usually followed, with the slope and speed of the treadmill increased at 3-minute intervals. Heart rate, blood pressure and ECG are monitored continuously. Exercise is continued until the patient asks to stop, or until the predicted maximum heart rate is achieved, or until significant ischaemia is demonstrated on the ECG.

OVERVIEW AND INDICATIONS

The exercise or stress test provides a great deal of information about cardiac function.

- What limits the patient's exercise capacity – chest pain, breathlessness, fatigue or orthopaedic problems? Is anxiety a major problem?

- Can the patient achieve an appropriate increase in heart rate and blood pressure with exercise? The 'target' heart rate is usually taken as 220 minus the patient's age in years. Patients who fail to achieve this target, and whose blood pressure does not rise, probably have impaired left ventricular function.

- If chest pain is the problem, can it be reproduced on the treadmill? If it can, is it accompanied by ischaemic changes on the ECG?

- Does exercise induce cardiac arrhythmias?

Because exercise testing done properly provides a lot of information, it should be supervised only by specially trained personnel. Furthermore, because it can produce arrhythmias (anything from ventricular extrasystoles through atrial fibrillation to ventricular tachycardia and ventricular fibrillation), two trained people who are skilled at resuscitation must be present. Cardiac arrests occur in about 1 in 10 000 tests.

Provided that fully trained technicians are present there is no need for a doctor, although medical help must be available nearby. Exercise testing takes at least 30 minutes, and including preparation of and explanation to the patient, probably longer than this. Most hospitals can scarcely provide for their own needs, and it is unlikely that direct-access exercise testing will ever become widely available.

POTENTIAL FINDINGS

- Most exercise testing is performed to aid the diagnosis of chest pain, or to assess the severity of angina if the diagnosis is already established. Various ECG 'abnormalities' develop with exercise, but a diagnosis of ischaemia can be made with confidence if there is 2 mm of horizontal ST-segment depression in any lead.

- The accuracy of exercise testing as a diagnostic tool depends on the type of patient being studied, but roughly speaking it is 80–90% accurate. In other words, there is still a 10% chance that a patient with intermittent chest pain has angina even when the exercise test has demonstrated no clear abnormality.

- Patients who have angina during the first two stages of the Bruce protocol (i.e. within less than 6 minutes of exercise) probably need a coronary angiogram. Those who cannot complete three stages (9 minutes) cannot hold a professional driving licence. Patients who can exercise for more than 9 minutes are unlikely to have severe coronary disease, but this is not always the case.

RELATED INVESTIGATIONS

- Patients who have an ischaemic ECG at rest and chest pain that sounds like angina need an exercise test only to assess the severity of their problem. It is not necessary to establish the diagnosis.

- An exercise test does not have the same function as a coronary angiogram. Exercise testing studies function, whereas angiography studies anatomy. Many people have anatomical coronary disease that does not impair function, and the two tests always need to be interpreted together.

PATIENT ADVICE

- The patient will need to undress to the waist so that electrodes can be applied to the chest. Women should be advised to wear trousers, or at least a skirt rather than a dress; 'sensible' shoes or trainers should be worn.

- Unless advised to the contrary by the hospital, the patient should not take beta-blockers on the day of the test, as these prevent a rise in heart rate. It is best not to take any anti-anginal drugs other than short-acting glyceryl trinitrate (GTN) before the test.

GP ADVICE

- Because of the risk of arrhythmias, and because the test can occasionally induce a myocardial infarction, a consent form may be needed – and almost certainly will be if the test is to be supervised by a technician.

- The GP must indicate what information he or she wants from the investigation.

Ambulatory ECG recording

OVERVIEW AND INDICATIONS

Ambulatory ECG recording is used to investigate intermittent symptoms that sound as if they might be due to a cardiac arrhythmia. The technique is most widely used for the investigation of palpitations, but it can also help to elucidate the cause of a syncopal or dizzy attack. As with any investigation, the more likely an arrhythmia appears to be on the basis of the patient's description, the more useful an ambulatory recording is likely to be. Investigating patients with unconvincing stories is seldom helpful.

There are two basic techniques, namely continuous recording of the ECG for 24 hours and event recording. Continuous recording, sometimes called 'Holter' recording after its inventor, is appropriate when attacks are frequent (at least twice a week) or if they incapacitate the patient. Event recording involves the patient activating a simple ECG recorder during an attack. Event recorders are much smaller than 24-hour recorders, but some patients may find them difficult to use.

One of the main problems with ambulatory recording is that most of the known cardiac arrhythmias can occur in asymptomatic individuals with perfectly normal hearts. A recording of an 'abnormality' of the ECG is therefore only really useful if it was made at a time when the patient had symptoms.

It will help the cardiac department to decide which form of ambulatory recording is more appropriate if a full description of the patient's symptoms is given.

Twenty-four-hour (Holter) recording is suitable when:

- attacks occur at least twice a week;
- attacks involve dizziness or syncope, when the patient becomes incapacitated;
- when the patient is unable, either because of physical infirmity or due to anxiety, to activate an event recorder.

Event recorders should be used:

- when attacks occur once a week or less;
- when attacks last long enough (at least a few minutes) for the patient to make the recording;
- when the patient can understand and comply with the technique.

Most cardiac departments allow a patient to keep an event recorder for 3 or 4 weeks; attacks occurring less frequently than this may well never be recorded.

POTENTIAL FINDINGS

In a patient who complains of intermittent palpitations the most common findings are:

- sinus tachycardia (usually due to anxiety, but possibly due to a phaeochromocytoma);
- extrasystoles (supraventricular or ventricular);
- paroxysmal atrial fibrillation;
- other paroxysmal tachycardias.

In patients with syncopal attacks, recordings may show:

- bradycardias such as complete heart block;
- very fast arrhythmias such as ventricular tachycardia.

However, it has to be accepted that the vast majority of ambulatory ECG recordings find nothing abnormal at all.

RELATED INVESTIGATIONS

- A resting ECG should always be recorded first. First, it may show extrasystoles, which the patient will recognise as being associated with his or her palpitations, and then no ambulatory recording is necessary. Secondly, it may show that an unexpected arrhythmia (such as atrial fibrillation) is present all the time. Thirdly, it may show an abnormality such as the Wolff–Parkinson–White's syndrome (short PR interval plus widened QRS complexes), which makes the occurrence of a paroxysmal tachycardia likely.
- When ambulatory recording fails to detect any abnormality, it may help simply to give the patient an ECG request card and tell him or her either to come to surgery or to go to the hospital Cardiac or Accident and Emergency Department for an immediate ECG whenever the symptoms persist for long enough.

PATIENT ADVICE

- The patient needs to be told that the investigation is unlikely to help if they do not have symptoms while the recording is being made. They must keep a diary, noting the times at which symptoms occur.
- An ambulatory recorder measure about 15 × 10 × 5 cm and weighs one or

two pounds. It is worn on a belt around the waist (under the shirt if necessary). Event recorders are the size of a thick credit card and can be kept in the pocket or handbag until they are needed.

GP ADVICE

- The GP must realise that, on the whole, ambulatory recording is not very helpful. It is invaluable when the patient has symptoms sufficiently often that a recording can be made during an episode of palpitations or syncope, but in real life this does not often happen.

- The report on the recording will usually describe any arrhythmia accurately. However, it will not determine whether such an arrhythmia is within the limits of normality, or whether it should be treated. A GP who is presented with a report of what might be an important arrhythmia should probably seek cardiological advice before beginning treatment.

Cardiac catheterisation

DESCRIPTION

Cardiac catheterisation is performed under local anaesthesia, although a general anaesthetic may be used in children. The diameter of the catheters used is about 2 mm. The catheter is passed under X-ray control into the appropriate heart chamber, where pressure measurements are made and radio-opaque 'dye' is then injected. The dye can be visualised on a television monitor as it passes with the blood through the heart or coronary arteries, but a permanent cine-record is made at the same time. This record used to be in the form of film, but is now usually stored on compact disc. The right side of the heart (the right atrium, right ventricle and pulmonary artery) is approached by passing a flexible tube through a vein, and the left side (the left ventricle and the coronary arteries) is approached via a peripheral artery – usually, in both cases, the femoral.

OVERVIEW AND INDICATIONS

Cardiac catheterisation is performed:

- to measure pressures inside the heart; and
- to inject radio-opaque 'dye' that will outline structures such as the left ventricle and the coronary arteries – the correct term for this is angiography.

It is unusual to make pressure measurements without also performing an angiogram, and the term 'cardiac cath' is usually used to describe both.

Catheterisation of the right heart is usually performed in order to make pressure measurements for the assessment of mitral valve disease. Right-sided angiography is rarely needed, although it is sometimes used to investigate possible pulmonary embolism. Left heart catheterisation is needed for the assessment of aortic valve disease and for coronary angiography. Coronary angiography is essential for the assessment of angina if coronary artery bypass grafting (CABG) or percutaneous transluminal coronary angioplasty (PTCA) are contemplated, and this is now the main reason why cardiac catheterisation is performed.

POTENTIAL FINDINGS

The assessment of the severity of valve disease usually involves a combination of pressure recording and angiography, but coronary arteries are investigated by angiography alone. In either case, the records need to be processed and reviewed, and an immediate answer should not be expected.

The investigation will usually show whether or not intervention (valve replacement, CABG, PTCA) is necessary. If it is necessary, it will give a good indication of the likelihood of success and the risks involved.

RELATED INVESTIGATIONS

- Cardiac catheterisation provides different information to that obtained by the other cardiac tests, and must be regarded as complementary to the latter. Whereas an exercise test shows how the heart functions and how much pain the patient is experiencing, the angiogram will delineate structure, and it has to be remembered that just because an angiogram shows coronary disease it does not necessarily mean that this is the cause of a patient's symptoms.

- Echocardiography is nearly as accurate as cardiac catheterisation for the investigation of valve disease and left ventricular function, and in young people decisions about valve surgery may be taken on the basis of echo studies alone. In older people, however, it will usually be necessary to perform a coronary angiogram before surgery is contemplated, so catheterisation will be needed.

PATIENT ADVICE

- The investigation may be performed as a day case, or it may involve an overnight stay. Catheterisation is not painful, and there is no sensation as the catheters are passed to the heart. There is a feeling of flushing all over the body as the angiographic dye is injected. The patient should be told that the room will be darkened, but that they will be able to watch the progress of the test on the video monitor. At the end of the procedure it is necessary to press very hard on the groin for 20 minutes or longer to prevent bleeding.

- The main issue the patient must be informed about is the risk. Overall, the risk of a serious complication is about 1 in 700 cases. The risks mainly involve damage to the femoral artery as the catheter is inserted; there may be excessive bleeding, and aneurysms and false aneurysms may develop afterwards that require surgical repair. Damage to the aortic arch and coronary arteries can lead to a stroke or myocardial infarction. The risk of death from the procedure is about 1 in 2000 cases.

It is because of these risks that cardiac catheterisation is only undertaken when the ultimate benefit seems likely to be sufficient to outweigh them.

GP ADVICE

Because this is a potentially dangerous investigation, GPs should ask their specialist colleagues for an opinion, not for a cardiac catheter. There is a danger that specialists will feel that they must oblige by performing a catheter when they really feel that it is not indicated. This is not good medicine and it is not fair to the patient.

Ambulatory blood pressure recording

Portable recorders are available which measure blood pressure (BP) at pre-set intervals, usually once an hour. Patients do not find them comfortable, but they are reasonably accurate and they do provide a better record of a patient's BP than single recordings made even at daily intervals. Ambulatory recording is especially useful when a patient appears to develop high blood pressure when he or she sees a doctor (white-coat hypertension), but repeated records made by a practice nurse may be equally useful. Many patients now buy their own simple recorders and take their own BP daily, and this gives an overview which is nearly as useful as 24-hour recording.

The main problem with 24-hour ambulatory recording is that it produces a lot of data that are difficult to use. All of the hypertension trials are based on casual recordings, usually repeated two or three times, and it is not known what level of ambulatory BP should be treated. Is the peak pressure the important factor, or is it the average over the 24-hour period that matters? Should emphasis be placed on peak or average systolic or diastolic readings? Ambulatory recorders produce all of these figures, and more besides.

The most common findings of ambulatory recordings are that the patient's BP appears to be lower than expected, and that control seems to be adequate for most of the time.

Radionuclide investigations

Isotope (or radionuclide) studies are definitely for the specialist. They can be used to investigate left ventricular function, where they may provide slightly more information than echocardiography, but not much. They are more commonly used to look for exercise-induced ischaemia in patients where the ECG is unhelpful either because of conduction defects or due to previous infarction. Exercise tests are performed using an isotope of thallium, and the studies are often referred to as 'thallium tests'. From the patient's point of view they involve much the same procedure as an ordinary exercise test, although there is an intravenous injection of the isotope, and there has to be a long period of waiting between two periods of exercise so that reversible and irreversible areas of ischaemia can be differentiated.

Magnetic resonance imaging

MRI is undoubtedly the most important new investigation in cardiovascular disease. It can produce detailed non-invasive peripheral (but not yet coronary) angiograms, and it can detect venous thrombosis and pulmonary embolism. It can be used accurately to describe left ventricular motion, and blood flow through the myocardium can already be measured reasonably well.

From the patient's point of view, the tests are claustrophobic because they involve lying in a narrow, noisy tube for half an hour, but equipment is now under development that will make this unnecessary.

EAR, NOSE AND THROAT

Pure tone audiometry (PTA)

Vestibular investigations: caloric tests/
electronystagmography

Sleep investigations

Nasal/sinus endoscopy

Laryngoscopy

Needle biopsy

Radiological investigations for otological disease

EAR, NOSE AND THROAT

Brian O'Reilly

A wide variety of ear, nose and throat (ENT) investigations are performed in the out-patient setting, notably in the fields of audiometry, radiology and endoscopy. The increasingly ready availability of these investigations to GPs should not tempt the clinician to order tests which may be invasive, expensive or simply inappropriate. Before requesting any investigation, a clinician should be aware of its potential hazards and limitations, and above all have some idea of the possible results. It is rare for an investigation employed on a 'shot-in-the-dark' basis to produce a useful result; it is more likely to confuse the picture further and to arouse deep anxiety in the patient.

Pure tone audiometry (PTA)

DESCRIPTION

This is the fundamental test for any patient with a hearing loss or suspected middle or inner ear disorder.

It measures the threshold of hearing for each ear for the frequencies from 250 to 8000 Hz in 5 decibel (dB) steps. PTA is not a direct measure of an individual's ability to hear speech. For diagnostic purposes, the frequency range tested extends well above that of the human voice (250–3000 Hz), and the loss of speech discrimination may be quite disproportionate to the severity of loss demonstrated by PTA.

INDICATIONS

- Suspected hearing loss.
- Suspected middle or inner ear disorder.
- Speech delay in children.
- It is usually repeatable so can be used to monitor certain diseases objectively (e.g. otosclerosis, Ménière's disease).

POTENTIAL FINDINGS

- PTA distinguishes a 'conductive hearing loss' (due to external or middle ear causes) from a 'sensorineural hearing loss' (due to inner ear or intracranial causes).

- Although certain conditions produce a characteristic audiogram (e.g. Ménière's disease and noise-induced hearing loss), PTA alone is never diagnostic.

- It may indicate the need for further investigations (e.g. an MRI scan in cases of unilateral hearing loss).

RELATED INVESTIGATIONS

- **MRI** (see above).

- **Tympanometry**: this is a fast, simple and virtually risk-free investigation which requires only basic co-operation, so can be used for children of any age. It is almost but not absolutely diagnostic of 'glue ear'; wax or other external ear debris may produce a flat trace, as can a perforation or patent grommet (although these should record a higher compliance volume). The significance of a negative middle-ear presssure is variable. Ideally, tympanometry should be used in conjunction with clinical examination and an assessmnent of hearing loss.

- **Brain stem-evoked response audiometry (BSERA)**: this may be used for neurological investigation, but its principal role is in the investigation of suspected hearing loss in cases where a reliable PTA cannot be obtained. Compared to PTA it has the advantages that it is objective (so the patient cannot exaggerate his or her loss) and it can be performed under general anaesthetic (e.g. in infants). BSERA is most often used for the investigation of infants with suspected hearing loss (e.g. because of delayed speech development or repeated failure of screening tests). However, it is time-consuming and neither frequency-specific nor as sensitive as PTA.

PATIENT ADVICE

The examination is quick, non-invasive and readily accepted by most patients.

GP ADVICE

- There are several important technical limitations.

- Accuracy is dependent on the patient's willingness and ability to co-operate. A mental age of at least 3 years is usually required to produce a reliable result.

Exaggeration of the hearing loss is also possible, notably in compensation cases.

- A misleading result (usually an overestimate of the hearing loss) may also occur if the test is performed by an untrained audiometrician.

- The tests must be performed in a sound-proofed booth or at least in very quiet surroundings.

Vestibular investigations: caloric tests/ electronystagmography

DESCRIPTION

These remain the only means of testing each ear separately, so are still the mainstay of vestibular investigations. They involve a measured irrigation of the ears with warm and cool water (or occasionally air). Electrodes applied to the head (rather like an electroencephalogram, EEG) measure the action potential of the eye muscles generated by the nystagmus (electronystagmography – an objective measure).

INDICATIONS

- A suspected labyrinthine disorder.

- Occasionally indicated for a vestibulocochlear nerve or intracranial lesion when an MRI scan cannot be performed.

POTENTIAL FINDINGS

The most significant finding is a canal paresis, indicating reduced function of that vestibular apparatus. It does not indicate the cause or site of the lesion (i.e. the labyrinth, the vestibular nerve or the brainstem). Misleading results may arise from obstruction of one external canal, a middle-ear effusion or from natural suppression of nystagmus (e.g. in gymnasts).

RELATED INVESTIGATIONS

- The patient will usually require audiometry and will often need a scan and serology.

- Posturography tests, which directly and objectively test an individual's balance and are valuable in monitoring and assisting their rehabilitation.

PATIENT ADVICE

- Caloric tests will induce transient vertigo in patients with a functioning balance system. This is rarely severe and does not leave them unfit to drive.
- Any vestibular sedative should be discontinued at least 48 hours before the test.
- Patients with perforated eardrums or obstructed ear canals are excluded.

GP ADVICE

- Vestibular tests are only of value in the context of the patient's history, clinical signs and other investigations.
- Direct referral for these investigations is unlikely to be accepted by audiology departments.
- In the event of an acute attack of vertigo, the tests should be deferred at least until the patient is ambulatory.
- An active otitis externa or accumulation of wax in one or both ears will render the patient unfit for caloric tests.
- Complications of caloric tests are rare, but otitis externa is possible.

Sleep investigations

DESCRIPTION

These investigations involve observation of (at least) the following throughout the night:

- duration and frequency of apnoeic episodes;
- blood oxygen levels;
- pulse rate.

INDICATIONS AND POTENTIAL FINDINGS

Obstructive sleep apnoea (OSA) has gained increasing recognition as a potentially serious condition. The indications for sleep studies are as follows:

- snoring in association with apnoeic episodes;
- daytime hypersomnolence – which should be investigated.

Investigation of OSA in children is straightforward, as almost all cases are the result of obstruction by enlarged tonsils and/or adenoids. In adults, sleep studies confirm the diagnosis and assess its severity. For potential findings, *see* 'Description' above.

RELATED INVESTIGATIONS

- In children, a soft-tissue, lateral skull X-ray for adenoidal hypertrophy and narrowing of the postnasal airway.

- In adults, fibre-optic laryngoscopy, which may be performed with a short-acting hypnotic in an attempt to mimic sleep.

PATIENT ADVICE

- This painless investigation is usually carried out in a separate hospital room. Although many patients believe that they sleep poorly in these circumstances, the results generally contradict this.

- Adults should attend their initial out-patient appointment with their partner to give a full history.

GP ADVICE

In practice, many cases of OSA present with snoring as their major complaint and may seek referral for investigation and treatment of this alone. These cases will still require fibre-optic laryngoscopy and, depending mainly on their history, a sleep study may also be indicated.

Nasal/sinus endoscopy

DESCRIPTION

The endoscope allows a clear and magnified view of all parts of the nose and the sinus openings. For the first time, a clinical diagnosis of sinusitis can be made or excluded with confidence, and small tumours and early polyposis can be detected with ease.

INDICATIONS

- Chronic or recurrent facial pain associated with rhinorrhoea or nasal congestion.
- Facial pain associated with a bloodstained discharge.

- Clear, unilateral rhinorrhoea suggesting a cerebrospinal fluid (CSF) leak.

POTENTIAL FINDINGS

Endoscopy will reveal possible inflammation, tumours or structural abnormalities of the nose or sinuses.

RELATED INVESTIGATIONS

- **Allergy tests:** with the rising incidence of atopic diseases, the importance of identifying allergens is increasing. The methods available are the radioallergen serum test (RAST) and skin tests.
- Radiological investigations, such as sinus X-rays and X-rays of nasal bones, are of little value.
- **Computerised tomography (CT) of sinuses:** these are extremely valuable in the following situations: suspected chronic sinusitis (the scans will demonstrate even minor degrees of mucosal disease and anatomical abnormalities within the nose and sinuses); suspected nasal or sinus tumour; facial fractures (e.g. of the skull base or orbit).
- **MRI scans of the sinuses:** the appropriate sequences will highlight any sinus disease (inflammatory or malignant). Although it is more sensitive than CT and capable of greater soft-tissue differentiation, it has the disadvantage of being unable to demonstrate directly the bony anatomy of the sinuses, and still cannot be used to make a definite pathological diagnosis.

PATIENT ADVICE

- Nasal endoscopy is usually performed after the application of a topical anaesthetic which may leave the throat numb for about an hour, during which time the patient should not eat or drink.
- The examination is quick and safe and produces minimal discomfort, so is often performed as part of a routine rhinological examination, although patients may be referred specifically for it.

Laryngoscopy

The larynx is the commonest site of cancer in the head and neck, but tumours detected early have a fairly good prognosis whether they are treated by radiotherapy or surgery. The common out-patient methods are as follows.

- **Indirect laryngoscopy**: this is the oldest and simplest form of the investigation. It requires only basic equipment, but does need a co-operative patient and an experienced examiner.
- **Fibre-optic laryngoscopy**: since the endoscope is passed through the nose after application of a topical local anaesthetic, discomfort and gagging are rarely a problem. The examination can even be performed on infants with sedation.
- **Direct laryngoscopy**: a rigid endoscope provides potentially the best view of the larynx in a conscious patient, but again patient tolerance and examiner experience are essential.

Although any of these investigations may be uncomfortable, none of them is painful or hazardous. A topical anaesthetic may be used, in which case eating and drinking should be avoided until sensation has been restored to the throat.

INDICATIONS

- Over 2 weeks of hoarseness, particularly in smokers.
- Upper airway obstruction indicated by stridor or respiratory distress. In contrast to asthma, there will be inspiratory obstruction.
- Dysphagia.
- Persistent, enlarged cervical nodes. These may arise from a malignancy in the upper airway.
- Chronic or intermittent dysphonia. Although this is unlikely to arise from a malignancy, it is often treatable by speech therapy or surgery, especially with early intervention.

Needle biopsy

Most patients will readily undergo needle biopsy without anaesthesia, and there is little risk associated with the procedure. However, it does have significant limitations.

- Obtaining an adequate specimen for cytology requires some practice (or luck!).
- The results alone may not be helpful (e.g. secondary deposits of carcinoma in a lymph node do not reveal the site of the primary tumour).
- The results can be misleading, notably in parotid tumours.

INDICATIONS

- Any persistent (more than 3 weeks) swelling of the head or neck.
- Neck swelling associated with altered voice or swallowing.
- Evidence of malignancy (e.g. skin tethering, pain, facial nerve palsy).

Radiological investigations for otological disease

Plain X-rays are of little value in the investigation of otological disease, and they have been almost entirely superseded by CT and MRI scans. CT scans can be of great value in demonstrating abnormalities of the middle ear in the following situations:

- congenital deformities;
- chronic infection/cholesteatoma;
- trauma.

The scan is fast, harmless and painless. It needs to be of high definition with 'bone windowing', so the request must make the GP's suspicions clear.

MRI scans are ideal for detecting intracranial tumours such as acoustic neuromas. The indications for MRI are as follows:

- unexplained, unilateral (or asymmetrical) sensorineural hearing loss;
- sudden sensorineural deafness;
- new diagnoses of probable Ménière's disease (5% of these cases will turn out to be acoustic neuromas).

MRI scans are radiation-free, but may involve the injection of the paramagnetic substance gadolinium. Patients who suffer from claustrophobia may not be able to tolerate the confined space and noise of the equipment.

Radiology, MRI, CT, ultrasound and isotope scans can all provide valuable information about head or neck swellings. The choice of which, if any, of these techniques to use depends both on clinical suspicion and on their availability. Usually it is better to refer the patient for an urgent clinical opinion rather than waste valuable time on trials of antibiotics.

ENDOCRINOLOGY

Glucose tolerance test (GTT)

Thyroid imaging

Endocrinology

Michael Laker

Laboratory and imaging assessments of endocrine function are widely available by direct access. Biochemical investigations of endocrine function fall into two main groups, namely the collection of a single blood test, or a dynamic function investigation when multiple blood samples are collected in order to assess the secretion of hormones when their controlling mechanisms are challenged either by stimulation or by suppression. The latter investigations often involve venous cannulation and are best undertaken as an out-patient or in a programmed investigation unit. The glucose tolerance test (GTT) is a simple dynamic function test, and as it does not involve cannulation it can be performed in primary care.

Glucose tolerance test

DESCRIPTION AND INDICATIONS

The GTT is diagnostic for diabetes mellitus, although it is not required in the majority of cases, the diagnosis being made on the basis of clinical features together with evidence of hyperglycaemia. Diabetes is present if a fasting value exceeds those shown in Table 1, or if a random blood glucose concentration exceeds 11.1 mmol/L in plasma from a venous blood specimen or 10.0 mmol/L in whole blood collected following a fingerprick. Under these circumstances a GTT is not indicated. This is true provided that no other serious medical conditions which may reduce glucose tolerance are present, such as myocardial infarction, trauma or serious infection. However, a GTT should be carried out if any of the following are found:

- equivocal blood glucose concentrations;
- unexplained glycosuria in pregnancy;
- clinical features of diabetes with normal blood glucose concentrations.

POTENTIAL FINDINGS

See Table 1.

Table 1   Oral glucose tolerance test: diagnostic criteria for diabetes mellitus and impaired glucose tolerance in adults

	Plasma		Whole blood	
	Venous	Capillary	Venous	Capillary
Diabetes mellitus				
Fasting blood glucose (mmol/L)	≥7.8	≥7.8	≥6.7	≥6.7
2-hour blood glucose (mmol/L)	≥11.1	≥12.2	≥10.0	≥11.1
Impaired glucose tolerance				
Fasting blood glucose (mmol/L)	≤7.8	≤7.8	≤6.7	≤6.7
2-hour blood glucose (mmol/L)	7.8–11.1	8.9–12.2	6.7–10.0	7.8–11.1

PATIENT ADVICE

- The standard oral glucose tolerance test (OGTT) involves administering an oral glucose load of 75 g or its equivalent as partial starch hydrolysates.

- It is given in the morning after a fast of 10–16 hours.

- The subject should have been on a normal diet for at least the previous 3 days, and should not be suffering from any other acute medical condition.

- The test is carried out with the subject seated; smoking is not allowed during the test.

- The sugar load is dissolved in 250–300 mL of water which should be drunk by the patient within 5 minutes.

- Blood samples are collected both fasting and after 2 hours.

Thyroid imaging

Radionuclide and ultrasound scanning are the main imaging techniques used to investigate the thyroid gland, although CT scanning may be useful in cases of retrosternal goitre. The main reason for imaging the thyroid gland is to determine the nature of a thyroid nodule.

1 Radionuclide scanning

DESCRIPTION AND INDICATIONS

Radionuclide scanning is based on the principle that some radioactive isotopes are concentrated differentially in the thyroid gland, and that the pattern of accumulation may be visualised using a gamma camera. This allows the differentiation of functioning and non-functioning tissue. Pertechnate (99Tcm) is generally preferred to iodine for this purpose, as it is not modified biochemically by the gland. In addition, it has a short half-life (6 hours) and diffuses rapidly out of the gland, thus limiting the amount of radiation. The main indication is in the differential diagnosis of a solitary thyroid nodule.

POTENTIAL FINDINGS

Occasionally, a nodule is functioning and concentrating isotope, such nodules being benign adenomas. Adenomas function independently of the pituitary gland, and if pituitary secretion of thyroid-stimulating hormone (TSH) is suppressed, the remainder of the gland will show reduced isotope uptake. Most solitary nodules do not take up isotope; the differential diagnosis includes a cyst, adenoma or carcinoma.

RELATED INVESTIGATIONS

Ultrasound and fine-needle aspiration biopsy (see below).

PATIENT ADVICE

Radionuclide scanning is relatively simple to perform. No special preparation is required, the isotope being administered intravenously, and thyroid tissue is visualised after 20 minutes using a gamma camera.

2 Ultrasound

Ultrasound scanning of the thyroid is used in the differential diagnosis of a thyroid nodule, and is a simple technique which requires no special preparation. Ultrasound normally produces a pattern of fine echoes, and the technique determines whether a nodule is cystic, solid, or a mixture of cystic and solid components. A cystic lesion is unlikely to be malignant, although a solid lesion may be an adenoma or a carcinoma. Both solid and cystic lesions should be further investigated by fine-needle aspiration biopsy and cytological examination of the aspirate.

GASTROENTEROLOGY

GASTROENTEROLOGY

Atul Sinha and Jeremy Nightingale

There are many investigations that test for abnormalities of gastrointestinal structure and/or function. The availability of such tests is largely determined by locally agreed guidelines. These in turn depend on the local prevalence of an illness, the cost, and the expertise available to perform the investigation. Gastrointestinal investigations can be divided into the following categories: endoscopic investigations; imaging tests; liver biopsy; *Helicobacter pylori* testing; motility studies; manometry; pH studies; and absorption tests.

Endoscopic investigations: overview

These include oesophagogastroduodenoscopy (OGD), enteroscopy, colonoscopy, sigmoidoscopy and proctoscopy. Endoscopic retrograde cholangiopancreatography (ERCP) and endoscopic ultrasound require both endoscopic and radiological skills, and are discussed in the section on imaging tests. The tests all involve direct visualisation of the gastrointestinal lumen with a flexible fibre-optic endoscope.

GP ADVICE (GENERAL)

NB For GP advice specific to each particular type of endoscopy, see the relevant section.

Complications may relate to the procedure (e.g. perforation or haemorrhage) or to the sedation given (e.g. hypoxia, aspiration, cardiac dysrhythmias and/or drug reactions). The risks are greater in elderly patients and in patients with concurrent illnesses (e.g. ischaemic heart disease or chronic obstructive pulmonary disease).

When requesting a test it is important to give the endoscopist as much information as possible for patient safety, and to ensure that the endoscopist looks carefully for the suspected lesion and takes appropriate biopsies. For example, if a patient is anaemic, duodenal biopsies will need to be taken to look for evidence of coeliac disease. Patients with diabetes mellitus should omit their morning treatment and must be the first patients on a morning endoscopy list. If a patient is taking warfarin and biopsies are required, the patient should stop warfarin for at least 2 days before the procedure, and heparin will be used to cover the procedure. Patients with previous endocarditis, prosthetic heart valves, surgically constructed pulmonary shunts and/or synthetic vascular grafts less than 1 year old all require antibiotic prophylaxis before any endoscopic procedure. No antibiotic cover is given to protect orthopaedic or any non-vascular related prostheses. It is helpful to have a knowledge of previous abdominal surgery. Most endoscopists avoid (except in an emergency) endoscoping pregnant women or patients within 6 weeks of a myocardial infarction.

PATIENT ADVICE (GENERAL)

NB For patient advice specific to each particular type of endoscopy, see the relevant section.

Following endoscopy, patients who have had sedation cannot drive and must not operate machinery; they will also need someone to take them home. They will have impaired memory and may not remember the procedure or its findings. They should also have a contact telephone number to ring if any problems occur.

1 Oesophagogastroduodenoscopy

DESCRIPTION

An OGD may be performed by doctors or by nurse endoscopists. A small dose of benzodiazepine (midazolam or diazepam, 2.5–10 mg IV) may be given. The oesophagus, stomach and duodenum (to the third part) are examined. The procedure allows biopsies to be obtained and therapeutic procedures such as injection sclerotherapy, banding of varices or placement of oesophageal stents to be performed.

INDICATIONS

- In patients aged under 45 years, an endoscopy may be considered if there is persistent dyspepsia that is unresponsive to conventional therapy.
- In those aged over 45 years with a recent onset of dyspepsia, an endoscopy is recommended (BSG Dyspepsia Guidelines, 1996).
- Weight loss, anorexia, iron-deficiency anaemia, suspected malabsorption or gastrointestinal bleeding might all merit an endoscopy, especially if associated with dyspepsia.
- Patients with heartburn should be endoscoped if they have dysphagia or weight loss, and at least once if they are over 45 years old to detect a Barrett's oesophagus.

- Patients with a Barrett's oesophagus are endoscoped annually with multiple biopsies being taken to detect premalignant or early malignant changes.

POTENTIAL FINDINGS

- Many gastro-oesophageal problems may be diagnosed, from hiatus hernia to ulcers, tumours or coeliac disease.
- *Helicobacter pylori* infection may be diagnosed by urease testing of a gastric biopsy.
- A normal endoscopy may be of value for reassuring an anxious patient.

RELATED INVESTIGATIONS

- Patients with high dysphagia should have a barium or Gastrograffin swallow before an endoscopy, because there is a dangerously high perforation risk during endoscopy for high dysphagia. A Gastrograffin swallow can differentiate obstructive lesions from motility disorders, and serves to warn the endoscopist of potential problems.
- Sometimes patients with acid reflux have a normal endoscopy. This does not mean that they do not have reflux, but merely that no macroscopic oesophageal damage has occurred. A 24-hour pH study of the oesophagus may be performed to confirm this situation.

PATIENT ADVICE

- The patient should have nothing to eat or drink for 4–6 hours before the endoscopy.
- At the time of the procedure the throat is sprayed with lignocaine, and as this may cause difficulty in swallowing, the patient cannot eat or drink for half an hour after the procedure.

GP ADVICE

- If this is the patient's first diagnostic endoscopy, they should stop proton-pump inhibitors and H_2-antagonists for at least 1 week before the procedure, as these drugs may heal inflammation/ulcers so that the endoscopy does not show the cause of the symptoms.
- The likelihood of a complication needing hospital admission is about 1 in 1000 cases, and that of death is 1 in 10 000 cases.
- Occasionally, retching during the procedure can induce a Mallory–Weiss tear.

- It is normal for the patient to complain of soreness in the throat for a few hours after the procedure.
- The presence of subcutaneous emphysema in the neck and supraclavicular areas should arouse the suspicion of oesophageal perforation.

NB For general GP and patient advice for endoscopy, see the Overview section above.

2 Colonoscopy

DESCRIPTION

A colonoscopy involves the examination of the whole colon (usually 90 cm of scope is used) and often the terminal ileum. In general, men are easier to colonoscope than women, as there is less abdominal space and thus less looping of the scope.

INDICATIONS

- After a barium enema has shown a probable abnormality.
- When an OGD has been normal in the investigation of iron-deficient anaemia.
- When a flexible sigmoidoscopy has shown one or more left-sided colonic polyps.
- In the event of diarrhoea, abdominal masses or terminal ileal abnormalities.
- Surveillance colonoscopies are performed every 2 years for patients who have had ulcerative colitis that has extended from the rectum to beyond the hepatic flexure for more than 10 years.
- Patients with a family history of colon cancer (two or more first-degree relatives), especially if it presented in a relative under 45 years of age.
- Patients who have had high-risk polyps (larger than 1 cm in size, three or more, or with a tubulovillous or severely dysplastic histology). Such patients are screened every 3 years.

POTENTIAL FINDINGS

- Colonoscopy is useful for diagnosing a wide range of colonic disease, including inflammatory bowel disease, polyposis and colonic cancer.
- Incidental findings may include diverticular disease and melanosis coli, which is due to chronic laxative abuse and gives the colonic mucosa a dark pigmentation.

RELATED INVESTIGATIONS

A double-contrast barium enema is nearly as sensitive as colonoscopy in detecting small lesions, and has a smaller risk of causing discomfort or complications. However, it does involve radiation exposure and biopsies are not obtained.

PATIENT ADVICE

- Colonoscopy does cause discomfort, especially if there has been a previous abdominal hysterectomy or other abdominal surgery, or if there is severe diverticular disease.
- Iron preparations should be stopped 3–4 days before colonoscopy.
- The patient should have no indigestible or high-fibre food for 24 hours prior to the procedure.
- The bowel is cleared with either a stimulant or osmotic laxative and a large oral fluid intake. An additional enema may be administered 1 hour prior to the procedure.
- The patient will be sedated with a benzodiazepine and an opiate analgesic.
- The procedure usually takes 30–45 minutes.

GP ADVICE

- Most people feel bloated after a colonoscopy, due to the air that is inserted.
- There is a small risk of the large bowel being perforated (1–2 in 1000 cases), and this may need surgery that can result in a temporary ileostomy or colostomy. Bleeding is less common (1 in 1000 cases). Both of these complications are more likely if a polyp is removed.
- Closed perforation due to full-thickness heat damage to the bowel wall may not be apparent for a day or two after the procedure. The patient may experience localised abdominal pain and fever, and examination may reveal signs of peritonitis.
- The risk of death from a colonoscopy is 1 in 10 000 cases.

NB For general GP and patient advice for endoscopy, see the Overview section above.

3 Flexible sigmoidoscopy

DESCRIPTION

A flexible sigmoidoscopy examines the left colon and often the distal transverse colon using a 60-cm-long scope.

INDICATIONS

The most common reasons for performing a flexible sigmoidoscopy are to investigate rectal bleeding and diarrhoea.

POTENTIAL FINDINGS

These are the same as for a colonoscopy.

RELATED INVESTIGATIONS

A flexible sigmoidoscopy is often performed in conjunction with another investigation – with a proctoscopy for rectal bleeding in which the blood is separate from the stool, and with a double-contrast barium enema if the blood is mixed in with the stool.

PATIENT ADVICE

- A phosphate enema is given 20–30 minutes prior to the procedure.
- The procedure takes 5–15 minutes and sedation is not usually needed.

GP ADVICE

The complications are the same as for a colonoscopy, but less frequent.

NB For general GP and patient advice for endoscopy, see the Overview' section above.

4 Proctoscopy

DESCRIPTION

After a digital rectal examination, a proctoscope (a rigid tube with a light attached) is inserted through the anus, the patient is asked to strain, the tube is then withdrawn slowly and haemorrhoids are looked for. If found, they can be injected or banded.

INDICATIONS

Rectal bleeding, especially if blood is fresh and separate from the stool.

POTENTIAL FINDINGS

Haemorrhoids, anal fissure or anterior mucosal prolapse.

RELATED INVESTIGATIONS

Sigmoidoscopy (see above).

PATIENT AND GP ADVICE

- Usually no preparation is required, but if the bowel is full of stool a phosphate enema may be given.
- Complications are rare, except when haemorrhoids have been injected or banded.

5 Enteroscopy

This procedure is only available in a few specialised centres, and it involves the patient swallowing a video-enteroscope 170–250 cm in length, which on withdrawal can examine the proximal small bowel. It is mainly used for patients with obscure gastrointestinal bleeding, investigation of suspected small-bowel Crohn's disease and the evaluation of abnormal small-bowel radiology. The procedure lasts 30–45 minutes.

Imaging tests

1 Barium swallow

DESCRIPTION

This involves the patient drinking barium or Gastrograffin, and the progress of the latter down the oesophagus being monitored with cineradiography or videofluoroscopy. It provides information about the morphology and motility of the oesophagus.

INDICATIONS

- Oropharyngeal dysphagia (due to abnormalities affecting the pharynx and the upper oesophageal sphincter).
- Dysphagia when an OGD has been normal.
- A patient who is intolerant of OGD or an operator who is unable to pass a scope.
- To assess an oesophageal leak (e.g. perforation or tracheo-oesophageal fistulae).
- Rarely, to assess reflux symptoms or retrosternal pain.

POTENTIAL FINDINGS

- Oesophageal dysmotility (achalasia, diffuse spasm, nutcracker oesophagus and tertiary oesophageal contractions).
- Hiatus hernia and reflux.
- Pharyngeal pouches and oesophageal diverticulae.
- Oesophageal and pharyngeal tumours or strictures.
- Oesophageal varices.

RELATED INVESTIGATIONS

Oesophagogastroduodenoscopy (see above).

PATIENT ADVICE

The patient is usually asked to fast overnight prior to the procedure.

GP ADVICE

Aspiration of contrast may occur. If this is likely (e.g. due to oesophageal perforation or post-operative assessment of surgical anastomoses), a water-soluble contrast agent (e.g. Gastrograffin) should be used.

2 Barium meal

DESCRIPTION

This involves swallowing a small amount of a gas-producing agent (bicarbonate), followed by a barium solution (occasionally Gastrograffin) to give double-contrast images. The patient is turned in order to coat the gastric lining evenly, and X-ray views of the stomach and duodenum are obtained. A smooth-muscle relaxant may be given intravenously.

INDICATIONS AND RELATED INVESTIGATIONS

The indications are essentially the same as for an OGD. A barium meal is administered in preference to an OGD only if the patient is intolerant of the latter, if the operator cannot gain access to all of the stomach and duodenum, or sometimes for suspected gastric outlet obstruction.

POTENTIAL FINDINGS

- Benign or malignant ulcers.
- Erosive gastritis.
- Benign lesions such as polyps.
- Gastric infiltration with malignancy.

PATIENT ADVICE

- The patient will need to starve for 6 hours prior to the procedure.
- The ingestion of bicarbonate may cause a short period of discomfort.

COMPLICATIONS

Barium can solidify if it remains in one part of the gut for a long period. It is also extremely irritant if it leaks outside the bowel. Thus when bowel obstruction or perforation is suspected, the less-irritant Gastrograffin is used as the contrast agent, although it does not give such clear images.

3 Barium follow-through (BaFT)/small-bowel enema (SBE)

DESCRIPTION

In a BaFT, barium is taken orally, metoclopramide is usually given intravenously to hasten gastric emptying and images of the small intestine are obtained. The patient may be turned and various pressures applied to the abdomen in order to separate bowel loops and obtain optimal images. This can be combined with a barium meal, but the agents used to help this slow gastric emptying and cause the barium to flocculate in the small bowel, so this combination is not recommended.

The barium can be given through an oro- or nasojejunal tube situated at the duodeno–jejunal junction (SBE).

INDICATIONS

- This investigation is usually performed when small-bowel Crohn's disease, small-bowel obstruction or a fistula is suspected.
- It may be used for unexplained gastrointestinal bleeding or to look for a small-bowel lymphoma in a patient with coeliac disease.

POTENTIAL FINDINGS

- Dilated bowel loops due to obstruction or ileus.
- Thickened mucosal folds due to inflammation.
- Strictures with proximal obstructive features (e.g. Crohn's disease or tuberculosis).

PATIENT ADVICE

The introduction of nasoduodenal tube may cause discomfort. However, many radiologists consider that the images from an SBE are better than those from a BaFT.

GP ADVICE

There is a small risk of perforation due to the guide-wire used in a small-bowel enema.

4 Barium enema

DESCRIPTION

Barium is introduced into the left colon through an enema catheter that is inserted into the rectum. Air is then gently pumped through the catheter and the patient is turned. These manoeuvres cause the barium to coat the remainder of the colon, giving a double contrast (air and barium). Abdominal and pelvic X-rays are taken in various views. A smooth-muscle relaxant may be used to reduce peristalsis and bowel spasm.

INDICATIONS AND RELATED INVESTIGATIONS

- This procedure is most commonly performed after a flexible sigmoidoscopy to check that the proximal colon is normal.

- Its indications are much the same as for a colonoscopy. It is usually done for patients with rectal bleeding/diarrhoea when a flexible sigmoidoscopy and proctoscopy have been normal. It is nearly as sensitive as colonoscopy in detecting small lesions, and has a smaller risk of causing discomfort or complications, but it does involve radiation exposure, and biopsies are not obtained.

- It may also be performed if a patient is intolerant of colonoscopy or if a complete colonoscopy cannot be undertaken (e.g. due to a stricture).

POTENTIAL FINDINGS

- Benign or malignant strictures with or without obstruction.

- Polyps and tumours.

- Diverticulae.

- Sigmoid volvulus.

PATIENT ADVICE

- The colon is prepared in a similar manner to that for colonoscopy.

- The procedure involves frequent changes of position, which may be difficult for elderly patients.

- Air insufflation of the colon is uncomfortable.

GP ADVICE

- There is a very small risk of colonic perforation during the procedure (about 1 in 25 000 examinations). Other complications include haemorrhage and vasovagal episodes.

- Good bowel preparation is critical.

- Patients with poor anal sphincter tone may be unable to hold the barium in the colon for long enough to allow the procedure.

- Patients who may be pregnant should not be given a barium enema.

- A combination of flexible sigmoidoscopy and double-contrast barium enema is often used (rather than a colonoscopy) to investigate colonic symptoms, as it is safer, quicker, less painful and often more easily obtainable.

- Biopsies and therapeutic procedures require a colonoscopy.

5 Ultrasound examination

DESCRIPTION

Ultrasound examination (with Doppler) is widely availabile, painless and safe. High-frequency sound waves are used to image the organs. This procedure can be used to assess the texture of organs, identify focal lesions, determine whether a lesion is liquid or solid, and assess blood flow within vessels. Endoluminal ultrasound probes are now available which can assess the oesophagus (used for assessing depth of tumour invasion) or pancreas (size of and structures involved in a pancreatic neoplasm).

INDICATIONS

- Ultrasound is the initial investigation used for a jaundiced elderly patient, as it will determine whether the jaundice is due to gallstones or a neoplasm.
- It can be used to check for many abdominal diseases (e.g. Crohn's disease, pancreatic or renal disease), to stage tumours, and to assess hepatic texture, portal vein flow and patency.
- Using ultrasound guidance, biopsies may be taken.

POTENTIAL FINDINGS

- Hepatic findings include cirrhosis, fatty infiltration, tumours or abscesses, portal vein thrombosis or Budd–Chiari syndrome.
- Other findings include gallstones, pancreatic abnormalities, thickened bowel wall, renal stones, and aortic, ovarian or uterine abnormalities.

PATIENT ADVICE

- The patient may be fasted for a few hours prior to the examination, to allow the gall-bladder to be full and the stomach empty.
- A full bladder is necessary for a pelvic ultrasound examination.
- The examination has no recognised complications.

6 Endoscopic retrograde cholangiopancreatography

DESCRIPTION

A side-viewing endoscope is passed into the duodenum and a catheter is introduced through the duodenal papilla into the biliary system or the pancreatic duct. Iodinated contrast is injected through the catheter and radiographs are obtained. A guide-wire can be introduced in a similar manner, over which instruments can be passed for various therapeutic procedures such as sphincter-otomy, stone extraction and stent placement. ERCP is a technically difficult procedure that depends on operator expertise, and it may not always be successful.

INDICATIONS

- Obstructive jaundice with dilated bile ducts shown on ultrasound examination (tumour or gallstones).

- Recurrent pancreatitis.

- Prior to a laparoscopic cholecystectomy if there are abnormal liver function tests or stones in the common bile duct (bile duct stones cannot easily be removed laparoscopically. They may be removed via ERCP so that a laparo-scopic rather than open cholecystectomy can then be used to remove the gall-bladder).

- Occasionally, the side-viewing endoscope is used to obtain histology or brushings from a pancreatic or biliary neoplasm.

- Most ERCPs are undertaken with a view to performing a therapeutic procedure (e.g. gallstone extraction with sphincterotomy or palliative biliary stenting).

POTENTIAL FINDINGS

- Obstruction of the bile duct or pancreatic duct by strictures or stones.

- Pancreatic or biliary malignancy.

- Sclerosing cholangitis.

- There may be a dilated biliary system without any obvious cause; this can occur after a cholecystectomy or after a gallstone has passed spontaneously.

- Chronic pancreatitis may be diagnosed.

RELATED INVESTIGATIONS

- Percutaneous trans-hepatic cholangiography (PTC) is performed by passing a small needle into the liver until it makes contact with a bile duct. Contrast is then introduced and images of the biliary tree are obtained. Most therapeutic procedures can be performed via the liver if ERCP has been unsuccessful (e.g. stenting, balloon dilatation of the ampulla).

- A CT scan may help with the diagnosis.

PATIENT ADVICE

- Preparation is similar to that for a gastroscopy.

- The procedure is uncomfortable, and intravenous sedation, strong analgesia and sometimes an antibiotic may be used.

- There is a risk of complications, especially with therapeutic procedures and in the elderly with concomitant illness.

- It may occasionally be necessary for the patient to stay overnight in hospital for observation following the procedure.

GP ADVICE

- The risk of death resulting from the procedure is about 1 in 1000 cases. The procedure has a 3% risk of causing pancreatitis in diagnostic procedures and an 8–12% risk for therapeutic procedures.

- There is a 2% risk of causing significant bleeding. Rarely, a perforation of the duodenum (< 1%) or infection of the bile ducts (cholangitis) may occur.

- Although most of the complications occur early (within 12 hours) after the ERCP, delayed bleeding, cholangitis and missed perforation need to be borne in mind. Gallstone ileus may occur as a result of passing gallstones into the small bowel following a sphincterotomy.

7 CT scanning

DESCRIPTION

This technique uses a rotating X-ray source and detectors to collect information which is then digitally processed to produce images of the body. Contrast scanning can be used to increase the sensitivity of the procedure.

INDICATIONS

- This procedure is used to investigate further abnormalities detected on ultrasound (e.g. focal hepatic lesions) and to stage malignancies (e.g. oesophageal, gastric, pancreatic and colorectal).
- CT scanning is particularly useful for visualising structures that are obscured by bowel gas.
- A CT scan may be used to guide a biopsy/aspiration needle.

POTENTIAL FINDINGS

- Diffuse disease involving abdominal organs (e.g. malignant infiltration).
- Focal lesions (e.g. abscesses, tumours and infarction).
- Lymph-node metastases and local invasion by tumour.

RELATED INVESTIGATIONS

- **MRI scanning**: this offers better soft-tissue differentiation, but is more expensive and not as widely available.
- **Spiral CT**: this recent development allows the X-ray tube and detectors to rotate continuously around the patient, rather than making just a few revolutions at a time as in conventional CT scanning. This improves the image obtained. It can be combined with contrast injection – both angiography and cholangiography (using agents excreted in the bile).

PATIENT ADVICE

- The procedure involves lying on a narrow table inside a large ring-shaped structure, and can produce a sense of claustrophobia.
- The patient will be asked to hold his or her breath for several seconds at a time in order to allow adequate exposures to be achieved.

GP ADVICE

- Any contrast allergy must be mentioned prior to the procedure.
- Pregnancy is a contraindication to abdominal CT scanning because of the radiation involved.

8 Magnetic resonance imaging

DESCRIPTION

This technique utilises the radio-frequency energy emitted by hydrogen nuclei in tissues, during magnetic relaxation after momentary radio-frequency excitation within a strong external magnetic field, to create an image of the tissue. This technique offers better soft-tissue resolution than CT scanning. Contrast scanning enhances the sensitivity still further.

INDICATIONS

Detection of soft-tissue tumours (mainly hepatic). It provides better soft-tissue differentiation than CT scanning, but is more expensive and less widely available.

PATIENT ADVICE

Claustrophobia may be a problem, despite sedation.

GP ADVICE

As the patient is exposed to a strong magnetic field, cardiac pacemakers, aneurysmal clips, early prosthetic heart valves, metallic foreign bodies in the eye and other implanted metallic objects are contraindications. Vascular stents and metallic prostheses are considered to be safe, but can make images difficult to interpret.

Liver biopsy

DESCRIPTION

Tissue can be obtained from the liver by either the percutaneous or the transjugular approach. Local anaesthesia is sufficient for percutaneous biopsy unless the patient is unco-operative, in which case sedation or even general anaesthesia may be required. A tiny, 1-millimetre cut is made in the skin over the liver and a special cutting or aspiration needle is passed into the liver to obtain a core of tissue. The patient holds his or her breath in expiration for a few seconds during the passage of the needle. After the procedure the patient is monitored closely for 4–6 hours before being discharged.

The transjugular approach is more difficult, but carries a smaller risk of bleeding. It can be performed even in the presence of ascites or severe emphysema. However, the size of the sample obtained is smaller than that obtained percutaneously. It is essential to obtain a coagulation profile and to perform blood grouping prior to the procedure. Liver biopsy is usually carried out under ultrasound guidance.

INDICATIONS

- Persistently abnormal liver function tests.
- Unexplained hepatomegaly.
- Suspected chronic hepatitis.
- Possible cirrhosis, infiltrative liver disease or tumours (primary or secondary).
- Screening of relatives of patients with disease (e.g. haemochromatosis).
- Before and after liver transplantation.

POTENTIAL FINDINGS

Many different diagnoses may be made according to the various histological, immunological, microbiological and biochemical tests that can be performed on the liver tissue.

PATIENT ADVICE

- The patient may be asked to fast for several hours before the procedure.
- Some degree of patient co-operation is essential for the procedure (e.g. holding their breath at the appropriate moment).
- There may be some pain.
- Occasionally, an overnight hospital stay for observation may be required.

GP ADVICE

- There is a mortality rate of 0.015%, which occurs mainly in those with abnormal livers. This figure has improved as a result of the widespread use of ultrasound.
- Significant bleeding occurs in 0.2% of cases, with delayed haemorrhage

occurring up to 2 weeks later. An intrahepatic haematoma is common but usually asymptomatic, although it can cause fever and pain. Intrahepatic arteriovenous fistulae occur in about 5% of cases, but are usually asymptomatic.

- Puncture of the gall-bladder or bile duct with biliary peritonitis is uncommon. Puncture of other organs (e.g. kidney) is rare.

Helicobacter pylori tests

The tests available can be divided into invasive tests (which use gastric biopsies obtained at endoscopy) and non-invasive tests. A false-negative result may be obtained if non-serological tests are performed within 1 week of taking proton-pump inhibitors, bismuth or antibiotics.

1 Invasive tests (based on gastric biopsies)

- Histology of antral biopsy with special staining for *Helicobacter pylori*. This has a sensitivity of 90% and a specificity of > 95% in detecting *H. pylori*.

- Rapid urease tests – some of these may be called a 'CLO' test from the time when *H. pylori* was known as a '*Campylobacter*-like organism'. They depend on urease produced by the organism hydrolysing urea to ammonia in a test medium, causing a pH change that is manifested as a change in the colour of an indicator dye from yellow to pink. The sensitivity is > 90% and the specificity is close to 100%.

- Bacterial culture is time-consuming, difficult and not a readily available test. It does provide 95% sensitivity and 90% specificity. It is useful for determining patterns of drug sensitivity (especially metronidazole resistance).

2 Non-invasive tests

- **Serology:** ELISA kits that detect anti-*Helicobacter* IgG antibody in blood are widely used. After proper local validation, the laboratory-based test kits offer an inexpensive, fairly sensitive (80–90%) and specific (80–90%) method of detecting *H. pylori*. Near-patient serological tests that can be used in the office setting give a result within 10–15 minutes. However, the low sensitivity and specificity of these tests detracts from their usefulness. As circulating antibodies to *H. pylori* persist in high concentrations for several months even after successful eradication, these tests only provide definite information about whether or not there has been a recent infection – not about the current state of infection.

- **Urea breath tests (UBT):** these tests are sensitive ($> 95\%$), specific (100%), safe and easy to perform. They depend on the production of ^{13}C- or ^{14}C-labelled carbon dioxide from the hydrolysis of labelled urea by urease-producing *H. pylori* in the stomach. The labelled carbon dioxide is detected in the expired air. ^{14}C is radioactive, so ^{13}C is most commonly used, but it is more expensive. The test is performed after a 6-hour fast. Breath samples are collected by the subject blowing through a straw into a test-tube. The patient ingests a fatty meal to delay gastric emptying, followed by labelled urea with orange juice. Further breath samples are collected after 30 minutes and analysed for ^{13}C or ^{14}C. A ^{13}C breath test is commonly used to determine whether *H. pylori* has been eradicated after triple therapy.

Motility studies

The purpose of these techniques is to assess the motility and peristaltic activity of the bowel. This information is of importance in diagnosing conditions such as achalasia cardia, gastro-oesophageal reflux disease, nutcracker oesophagus, gastroparesis and slow-transit constipation. Radiological techniques are commonly used, although some centres are developing radioisotopic techniques.

Radiological techniques use serial X-rays or cineradiography to track the progress of ingested radio-opaque markers through various parts of the gastro-intestinal tract. The most common application of this technique is the barium swallow or dynamic oesophageal motility study. Ingested radio-opaque markers ('shapes') that are visible on abdominal radiographs are used to determine colonic transit times.

Manometry

Solid-state pressure transducers mounted on catheters as well as perfused catheter systems are used to assess the pressures generated by propulsive and mixing peristaltic waves, as well as the resting tone of various regions (most commonly the oesophagus, although the duodenum and anal sphincter can also be studied). The maximum luminal pressure generated by the peristaltic wave, the sequential passage of the peristaltic wave over successive segments of the bowel, and the resting tone and relaxation of the sphincters are all studied. These tests require special equipment and expertise, and are not readily available. Barium studies are usually performed first.

Indications for oesophageal manometry include assessment of oesophageal function prior to gastro-oesophageal reflux surgery, diagnosis of achalasia and pseudo-achalasia, investigation of chest pain thought to be of oesophageal origin (e.g. nutcracker oesophagus and diffuse oesophageal spasm) and assessment of high dysphagia thought to be of neuromuscular origin.

Anorectal physiology involves inserting a balloon into the rectum and rapidly inflating and deflating it. This test, together with a full-thickness rectal biopsy, is used to diagnose Hirschprung's disease. In addition, the patient's pudendal nerve latency period can be measured by electrically stimulating the nerve. This helps to determine whether a neuropathic process is affecting the anal sphincter (e.g. from a traumatic labour).

pH studies

This involves ambulatory 24-hour monitoring of the oesophageal pH using a catheter-mounted, multi-channel pH sensor. This is positioned in the oesophagus such that one sensor is located 5 cm above the lower oesophageal sphincter and the others are situated more proximally. The assembly is connected to a small recording device attached to a belt around the patient's waist. The apparatus is left *in situ* for 24 hours while the patient goes about his or her normal daily routine. The percentage of time for which the oesophageal pH value is < 4 is used to indicate acid reflux. The normal value is 4–5%. Separate analyses of daytime and night-time episodes of reflux are also performed. The patient is instructed to keep a record of his or her symptoms over the test period, and the symptoms are correlated with changes in oesophageal pH.

Indications include reflux symptoms without any endoscopic evidence of oesophagitis, assessment of patients prior to anti-reflux surgery, persistent symptoms despite acid-suppression therapy (it may detect biliary reflux), refractory asthma or recurrent laryngitis.

Absorption tests

If a patient has suspected malabsorption, a screening test may be performed (e.g. butterfat test, triolein breath test). If abnormal, the finding is confirmed with a

3-day stool collection for stool weight (normal range is 200–400 g/24 hours) and faecal fat test. Various tests are available to distinguish pancreatic causes from intestinal causes of malabsorption. A Schilling test using labelled vitamin B_{12} (cobalamin) can be performed to define the cause of vitamin B_{12} deficiency (*see* Haematology chapter).

HAEMATOLOGY

Bone-marrow examination

Schilling test

HAEMATOLOGY

Henry G Watson

By far the most common investigation which brings patients to the attention of the haematology service is the full blood count. Abnormal parameters are flagged up by the automated counter and this may result in the generation of a blood film. The blood film is then interpreted in conjunction with the available clinical history, and in certain cases the reporting haematologist may contact the referring GP for a discussion on the telephone. The film report may give a definite diagnosis, or it may yield a differential diagnosis with suggestions for further appropriate investigations. Further, rapid referral of urgent cases to the appropriate consultant haematologist is usual because of the seamless nature of haematology care as a combined clinical and laboratory service. The film report and interpretation of less urgent cases is relayed to the GP, who is then faced with the problem of explaining the findings and the nature of any further investigations to the patient. In this chapter some details of these investigations will be outlined.

Bone-marrow examination

DESCRIPTION

Bone-marrow examination may include marrow aspirate and trephine biopsy, depending on the suspected diagnosis from the clinical features and the blood-film appearances. Marrow examination allows analysis of the cellularity, cell morphology and the architecture of the 'factory where blood cells are made'. The interpretation should take into account the other features of the case, including the results of other related investigations (e.g. immunophenotyping and cytogenetic or molecular analysis of cells).

INDICATIONS

- Investigation of peripheral blood cytopenias or cytosis.
- Investigation of certain abnormalities of peripheral blood morphology.
- Investigation of paraproteinaemia.
- Staging of lymphoma.

- Staging of neuroblastoma (children).

Trephine biopsy is especially indicated in the following situations:

- investigation of myeloproliferative disorders;
- staging of lymphoma;
- cases of suspected carcinomatous infiltration of the marrow;
- cases where hypoplastic or aplastic anaemia is suspected.

POTENTIAL FINDINGS

The bone-marrow report will normally comment on aspects of the morphology and then draw a likely conclusion, ideally reached in conjunction with the clinical history. The following will usually be mentioned in the report:

- the marrow cellularity;
- the observed pattern of cellular maturation and any significant deviation from normal (e.g. left-shifted maturation suggesting an excess of immature cells, or maturation arrest as seen in cases of drug-induced agranulocytosis);
- in addition, the appearance of the cells will be commented on and a statement about the process of haematopoiesis will be given (e.g. normal, dysplastic or megaloblastic);
- the presence of an excess of any cell population will be commented on (e.g. blasts in acute leukaemia or myelodysplastic syndromes, or plasma cells in myeloma). If an excess of blasts is present, then the reporter will consider the cellular morphology and suggest the cell lineage from which they have arisen;
- the presence of non-haematopoietic cells;
- iron stores and pattern of iron uptake by erythroid progenitors;
- the trephine report will comment on the amount and pattern of reticulin deposited in the marrow.

RELATED INVESTIGATIONS

- Cytochemistry of the marrow allows further delineation of the lineage of blast cells, but is becoming increasingly outdated as a technique.
- Immunophenotyping helps to establish the lineage and maturity of cells by looking at their pattern of cell surface and cytoplasmic antigen expression.
- Cytogenetics allows the detection of chromosomal rearrangements, some of

which are strongly associated with certain disease processes and give valuable information about treatment and prognosis.

- Recently, molecular analysis of malignant cells has been used to define clonality of disorders and to follow up high-dose treatments and bone-marrow transplant as markers of early disease relapse.

- Other bone-marrow findings may trigger a variety of other investigations.

PATIENT ADVICE

Details of the procedure are as follows.

- It is a 10-minute out-patient procedure.

- Marrow is usually taken from the posterior iliac spine of the pelvis.

- The majority of examinations are performed with local anaesthetic, but in certain cases a small dose of a benzodiazepine may be given.

- The patient may experience discomfort at the time of the examination, but this ceases as soon as the procedure is completed.

- Patients who have had only local anaesthetic may drive home immediately after the procedure. Individuals who require sedation may not drive home.

- Complications associated with bone-marrow examination are extremely rare.

GP ADVICE

- Very occasionally, bruising or sub-periosteal haematoma may result in local pain after bone-marrow biopsy.

- Very rarely, superficial skin infection may complicate the procedure.

Schilling test

DESCRIPTION

The Schilling test determines whether the patient is able to absorb vitamin B_{12} and, if not, the site of malabsorption. This is achieved by measuring the absorption of radiolabelled cyanocobalamin and cyanocobalamin–intrinsic factor complex. The principle on which the test is based is the fact that vitamin B_{12} can only be absorbed by a normally functioning small intestine if it is bound to intrinsic factor (IF), a protein that is produced by the gastric parietal cells.

Failure to absorb vitamin B_{12} may therefore either be corrected by IF (pernicious anaemia (PA)) or it may not (small intestinal disease).

INDICATIONS

Investigation of a low serum vitamin B_{12} concentration.

POTENTIAL FINDINGS

Low serum vitamin B_{12} levels are most often due to malabsorption in Western countries. Occasionally, vegans may present with low vitamin B_{12} due to malnutrition. The Schilling test may have three outcomes:

- normal vitamin B_{12} absorption;
- vitamin B_{12} malabsorption corrected by IF (PA or gastrectomy);
- vitamin B_{12} malabsorption not corrected by IF (small intestinal disease).

RELATED INVESTIGATIONS

Other tests performed in the course of investigation of a low vitamin B_{12} level (which itself is most likely to have been generated by the finding of a macrocytosis on a full blood count or in the course of investigation of neuropathy or dementia) may be conducted either concurrently with the Schilling test or following it.

Tests that confirm a diagnosis of PA include the following:

- anti-IF antibodies are found in 50% of cases of PA, but are 100% specific for PA if found in the context of a low vitamin B_{12} level. Therefore, in cases of a low vitamin B_{12} concentration with a positive anti-IF antibody, there is usually no indication for a Schilling test unless it is considered likely that the patient actually has a small-intestinal cause of vitamin B_{12} malabsorption;
- endoscopy to demonstrate gastric atrophy.

Tests that are used in cases of vitamin B_{12} malabsorption not due to PA include the following:

- tests of small-intestinal function;
- small-intestinal contrast studies;
- small-intestinal biopsy.

PATIENT ADVICE

- The patient should be told that tests are being performed to determine the cause of the low vitamin B_{12} levels.

- The test involves swallowing a capsule of vitamin B_{12} with a tiny radioactivity content.
- Simultaneously, an intramuscular injection of vitamin B_{12} will be administered.
- A complete urine collection for 24 hours is required.
- The result will be available in less than 1 week.
- The patient is extremely unlikely to experience any side effects.
- If the Schilling test suggests PA, no more invasive investigation is required.
- If the Schilling test suggests small-intestinal disease, then further investigations will be required.

GP ADVICE

- The test is more likely to provide accurate information if the patient's vitamin B_{12} stores have been replaced (by treatment) before the test.
- The commonest cause of a spurious or odd result is incomplete urine collection.

NEUROLOGY

Imaging investigations

Neurophysiological investigations

Other investigations

NEUROLOGY

Carolyn A Young

Specialist assessment of a patient with neurological symptoms proceeds through four stages:

- establishing that there is a neurological lesion;
- localising it;
- identifying its probable nature;
- advising on management.

The history and clinical examination are critical, and are interpreted with knowledge of neuroanatomy and disorders affecting the nervous system. Investigations are used to confirm a diagnosis, to exclude alternative causes and to assess severity.

Few secondary-care investigations in neurology are appropriate for direct primary-care access. Many of them are highly specialised and extremely dependent on clinical input for accurate interpretation. Several involve small risks of morbidity or mortality. The need for such tests must be assessed by the hospital doctor taking responsibility for the investigation, who will also ensure that the patient is aware of any risks and obtain informed consent as necessary. In addition, neurological investigations regularly detect asymptomatic abnormalities. Risks of misdiagnosis are clearly high, and are even greater for non-specialists who have less clinical experience and familiarity with the investigation in question.

Imaging investigations

1 Computerised axial tomography (CAT)

DESCRIPTION

CAT (or CT) scans are derived from a series of X-ray images recorded from various angles and then analysed by computer. Tomographic slices are printed, and slice thickness and orientation may be varied depending on the condition being investigated. The brain, spinal cord, optic nerves and orbit may be examined in neurological practice. Contrast enhancement may be given intra-venously or sometimes intrathecally by lumbar puncture.

INDICATIONS

These are wide-ranging, and include investigation of possible mass lesions (neoplastic or inflammatory) (*see also* the 'Potential findings' section below).

POTENTIAL FINDINGS

- Lesions have specific patterns of density change and enhancement that allow them to be interpreted as neoplasm, abscess and so on.

- Sometimes abnormalities are anatomical (e.g. ventricle size, atrophy or midline shift).

RELATED INVESTIGATIONS

Other radiological investigations (e.g. MRI, magnetic resonance angiography (MRA)) are described later in this chapter.

PATIENT ADVICE

- The body part to be scanned passes through the scanner while the patient lies on a moving table.

- The patient must keep still during scanning.

GP ADVICE

- The radiologist requires clinical information to determine the scan type and guide use of contrast. Contrast-enhanced scans are not routinely performed because of the small risk of allergic reactions, neurotoxicity or systemic toxicity. Slice orientation and thickness can be varied depending on the differential diagnosis.

- If recent cerebral infarction is suspected, contrast is often avoided.

- The request form should state whether the patient has a known allergy to iodine or previous contrast use.

- The normal concerns over radiation exposure in recurrent use and pregnancy apply.

2 Magnetic resonance imaging

DESCRIPTION

High-intensity magnetic fields and radio-frequency waves produce tomographic slices of brain or spinal cord. Different phases of scanning (T1, T2) give better definition to particular areas of the brain depending on their constitution, especially water content. Contrast enhancement is useful in cases where the blood-brain barrier is defective.

INDICATIONS

- These are wide-ranging as in CAT (see earlier).
- MRI is more informative than CAT in certain conditions (e.g. suspected multiple sclerosis, vascular malformations, spinal disease) and when imaging the posterior fossa and foramen magnum.

POTENTIAL FINDINGS

Particular patterns of signal change and enhancement in T1, T2 or specialised sequences give information about a wide variety of pathologies (see above section on CAT and Indications).

RELATED INVESTIGATIONS

Other radiological investigations, including MRA, myelography and angiography.

PATIENT ADVICE

- The set-up is similar to CAT, but MRI is noisier and more claustrophobic.
- Examination times are usually longer.
- Some patients experience a temporary reduction in hearing for a short period (less than 1 hour) after the test.

GP ADVICE

- MRI scanning may be unsafe in patients whose bodies contain any ferro-magnetic materials (e.g. plates, wires, vascular clips, prostheses, shrapnel) or any implants which might be electrically or magnetically activated (e.g. pacemakers).

- The risks of neurotoxicity, systemic toxicity or allergic reaction to contrast are very small.

3 Magnetic resonance angiography

DESCRIPTION

This consists of a special magnetic resonance sequence to demonstrate blood flow in vessels without the use of contrast.

INDICATIONS

MRA is used for the investigation of many types of cerebrovascular disease.

POTENTIAL FINDINGS

These include stenosis and abnormalities of vessel wall (e.g. dissections, arterio-venous malformations, aneurysms).

PATIENT ADVICE

This is similar to that for MRI (see above).

GP ADVICE

It should be remembered that MRA produces a physiological rather than radiological image. The results of MRA are highly dependent on the radiologist and radiographer and the settings of the equipment used. Radiology departments should validate their MRA results against conventional angiography before offering the investigation in routine clinical practice.

4 Angiography

DESCRIPTION

This consists of examination of blood vessels by contrast injected via a transfemoral catheter to carotid arteries.

INDICATIONS

Angiography is used for the investigation of cerebrovascular disease, especially subarachnoid haemorrhage.

POTENTIAL FINDINGS

Findings are similar to those for MRA, but angiography may detect aneurysms that are too small to be seen on MRA.

PATIENT ADVICE

There is an approximately 1% risk of permanent stroke (or death) and a 4% risk of transient neurological deficit. The risk may be higher in patients who have recently had a subarachnoid haemorrhage.

GP ADVICE

- Angiography may be performed as a day-case procedure with the patient discharged home after several hours of bed rest if they are well and further bleeding from the femoral artery has not occurred.
- The patient must immediately be re-referred to the investigating unit if a significant haematoma develops in the groin, or if there is significant bleeding.
- The foot pulses should be checked to ensure pressure from any haematoma is not occluding femoral artery flow.

5 Myelography

DESCRIPTION

Contrast is injected into the cerebrospinal fluid (CSF) to allow radiological definition of the spinal cord, nerve roots and foramen magnum region. The contrast is usually given by lumbar puncture, although the cervical route may be used to give better visualisation of the cervical area or to show the upper border of a spinal block.

INDICATIONS

Myelography is used for investigation of degenerative disorders of the spine, arteriovenous malformations and spinal tumours.

POTENTIAL FINDINGS

These are wide-ranging, including cord or root compression, and cord expansion in spinal tumours or cysts.

RELATED INVESTIGATIONS

- CSF may be taken when the lumbar puncture is performed for contrast injection.
- Follow-up CT may provide more detail. If a syrinx is suspected, follow-up CT may be delayed for several hours to allow contrast to enter the syrinx.

PATIENT ADVICE

The patient lies on a myelogram table, which is tilted to move the contrast while a series of X-rays is taken (*see also* section below on lumbar puncture). Adequate hydration before and after myelography minimises neurotoxicity from contrast, which is uncommon and short-lived, lasting from hours to a day.

GP ADVICE

- Myelography has been largely replaced by MRA.
- It remains necessary for those patients who cannot undergo or tolerate MRA, and it offers additional information in certain conditions (e.g. arteriovenous malformation).
- As with other contrast examinations, the radiographer must be informed of iodine allergy or any previous reaction to contrast. The usual contraindications in pregnancy apply.
- Spinal arachnoiditis after months or years occurred with older contrast media, which have been replaced by water-soluble agents.

6 Doppler/duplex ultrasound

DESCRIPTION

Ultrasound imaging and Doppler sonography of the carotid arteries is a safe, non-invasive examination. Its primary indication is estimation of the degree of stenosis of the vessels.

INDICATIONS

- Investigation of carotid transient ischaemic attack (TIA) or stroke.
- Also useful in the investigation of other vascular abnormalities such as carotid dissection or subclavian steal.

POTENTIAL FINDINGS

- Imaging allows the arterial wall to be visualised and Doppler flow studies measure the velocity of blood flow in systolic and diastolic phases of the cardiac cycle. These flow rates allow stenoses to be estimated. However, the relationship between velocity and stenosis varies between different machines, and each laboratory must 'calibrate' its ultrasound machine by a comparative study with angiography.
- Carotid dissection is associated with poor flow signal in the internal carotid with a characteristic 'to and fro' signal which may be diagnostic.

RELATED INVESTIGATIONS

- Angiography (often now magnetic resonance angiography) to confirm the degree of stenosis or occlusion, and to inform about the risk/benefit ratio of carotid endarterectomy in that individual.
- Brain imaging with CT or MRI to visualise haemorrhages or infarcts.
- Echocardiography to seek cardiac sources of emboli.

PATIENT ADVICE

The examination is free of risk or discomfort. It takes about 20 minutes.

GP ADVICE

This examination is very dependent on the expertise of the provider.

It is important to remember that many stenoses are asymptomatic, and that as yet the surgical treatment of asymptomatic stenosis is not of proven benefit. Non-specialists tend to overdiagnose TIAs and minor strokes, so referral should ideally be made to a unit which will give an opinion as to whether the neurological symptoms really are due to carotid ischaemia, as well as conducting Doppler studies or other tests as indicated.

Neurophysiological investigations

1 Electroencephalography (EEG)

DESCRIPTION

Spontaneous brain electrical potentials can be recorded over the scalp.

INDICATIONS

Investigation of epilepsy, encephalitis, disorders of consciousness, and rare disorders such as Creutzfeldt–Jakob disease (CJD) and subacute sclerosing pan-encephalitis (SSPE).

POTENTIAL FINDINGS

- Particular patterns of spikes or spike and wave may support a diagnosis of epilepsy.
- Generalised or focal slow waves may be seen in encephalopathies and encephalitis.
- Characteristic stereotyped slow-wave abnormalities may occur in conditions such as CJD and SSPE.

RELATED INVESTIGATIONS

- **Ambulatory EEG**: a prolonged record over 24 hours or longer for out-patients or in-patients, using portable equipment strapped to the body. The apparatus has an event recorder which the patient presses at the onset of an attack. Normal medication should be continued unless the doctor arranging the test states otherwise. In-patient stay allows the patient to be observed and has a greater margin of safety if anticonvulsants are reduced in order to increase the likelihood of detecting a seizure. Out-patients make a daily visit at a pre-arranged time for tape and battery change. Provided that they keep the equipment dry and undamaged they can engage in normal day-to-day activities during monitoring.
- **Telemetry**: similar prolonged recordings, often made over several days of in-patient stay with the EEG transmitted by cable or radio. The patient is advised to bring something to do, as they are essentially restricted to their room throughout the procedure.

- **Videotelemetry**: a single room is set up for simultaneous video and EEG recording. The technician will show the patient which areas of the room can be seen and reassure them that the videotapes are not stored. Simultaneous videos of the patient and the EEG are observed in the neurophysiology department and/or ward office.

PATIENT ADVICE

- Electrodes will be placed on the scalp. The jelly used to improve electrical contact makes the hair sticky (some departments provide hair-washing facilities for out-patient use).
- The patient should take their normal medications unless instructed otherwise by the doctor requesting the test, and should bring a full list of medications when they attend for their appointment.
- During the procedure, which takes about 60–90 minutes, the patient may be asked to watch flashing (stroboscopic) lights or to hyperventilate.

GP ADVICE

It is very important not to over-interpret EEG records. Most EEGs are interictal (i.e. performed between seizures, when people with epilepsy may have normal records). Conversely, people without epilepsy may have EEG abnormalities. A detailed description of attacks, including an eyewitness account, is essential.

2 Sleep studies

DESCRIPTION

Multi-parameter recordings during sleep may measure heart rate, EEG, eye movements, respiratory muscle activity, nasal air flow and oxygen concentrations.

INDICATIONS

- To investigate upper respiratory and neurological disorders in which symptoms and signs alter during sleep. Examples include sleep apnoea and advanced neuromuscular disorders.
- To investigate primary disorders of sleep (parasomnias), including narcolepsy.

POTENTIAL FINDINGS

- Nasal and oral air flow cease for periods during sleep apnoea. In obstructive forms, respiratory efforts continue, and with central non-obstructive forms there is hypoventilation.

- Patients with neuromuscular disorders may show hypoventilation and hypoxaemia when voluntary cortical respiratory mechanisms decrease during sleep.

PATIENT ADVICE

- Testing may last all day or overnight.

- The patient should attend in a relatively sleep-deprived state.

- During daytime testing is it important to contrast sleep and awake cycles, so it is helpful to have a companion and to bring something to do during the awake cycles.

- The hospital may provide a sleep diary to be completed for a few weeks before testing.

GP ADVICE

Interpretation is aided by a full medication list and any additional information on nocturnal snoring or restlessness.

3 Nerve conduction studies (NCS)

DESCRIPTION

Conduction velocity in peripheral nerves can be measured using surface electrodes.

INDICATIONS

To investigate disorders of muscle or peripheral nerves, including root lesions.

POTENTIAL FINDINGS

- Sensory action potentials show increased latency and reduced amplitude in sensory nerve disorders, such as carpal tunnel syndrome.

- Repetitive nerve stimulation may confirm a decremental response in the compound muscle action potential in conditions that show fatiguability (e.g. myasthenia gravis).

- Other information that may be obtained includes motor nerve conduction velocity and compound muscle action potential, which is reduced if the motor nerve or muscle is damaged.

RELATED INVESTIGATIONS

Electromyography (EMG) is often performed at the same visit unless two prolonged investigations are necessary, such as repetitive stimulation and EMG.

PATIENT ADVICE

- It will be necessary to expose the limbs for measurement, and the patient should dress accordingly.
- The limb must be warm.
- Both right and left sides are often measured, as asymmetry is atypical and may indicate abnormality even if the results all fall within normal ranges.
- The tests take 30–120 minutes to complete.

4 Electromyography

DESCRIPTION

Skeletal muscle produces different types of electrical activity in neurogenic and myopathic disorders. Examination of several muscles can show a pattern of involvement indicating damage to nerve roots (lumbar, sacral or cervical) or individual peripheral nerves. Regional changes may be seen in myopathic disorders.

INDICATIONS

Investigation of muscles that are denervated or myopathic.

POTENTIAL FINDINGS

Normal patterns are distorted in characteristic ways depending on the underlying pathology. For example, in denervated muscle, insertional activity is increased and there is spontaneous firing at rest (e.g. fasciculations or fibrillations). In myopathies, muscle is usually silent at rest (except in polymyositis and some destructive myopathies). Motor units show reduced amplitude, shorter duration and polyphasia as damage in the unit is patchy. Myotonic muscle has character-istic discharges on electrode insertion and muscle contraction.

RELATED INVESTIGATIONS

Muscle biopsy, which should be performed in a different muscle to that sampled by EMG.

PATIENT ADVICE

- The limbs must be exposed, so appropriate clothing should be worn.

- Needle electrodes are necessary, and some patients experience discomfort.

- Minor bruising may occur at the site of needle puncture.

GP ADVICE

- The GP making the referral must inform the neurophysiologist if the patient is anticoagulated. Testing is rarely possible if the international normalised ratio (INR) must remain above 3. It is preferable if anticoagulation can be temporarily suspended or reduced.

- The value of EMG is highly dependent on the skill and experience of the clinician. On the basis of presentation and examination, particular muscles are sampled. Several sites are tested in each muscle, but if the trace appears slightly unusual further sites will be tested in order to clarify any abnormality. If a given muscle is involved, the clinician uses his or her anatomical knowledge to determine which other muscles to test.

- Analysis of the total examination is not automated but relies on the clinician. Only a representative sample of the total trace is recorded and printed. Furthermore, some abnormalities have a characteristic sound which is recognised by the experienced operator but not recorded.

5 Evoked potentials (EPs)

DESCRIPTION

Evoked potentials, sometimes called evoked responses (ERs), consist of averaged EEG responses during a series of identical sensory stimuli. Interpretation requires assessment of waveform, amplitude and latency. Delay indicates a lesion in the sensory pathway which may be visual, auditory or somatosensory.

INDICATIONS

EPs may provide supporting evidence where history, examination, other investigations or knowledge of disease presentation suggest a particular pathway may be affected. Common examples include abnormal visual EPs in multiple sclerosis due to subclinical attacks of demyelination in the optic nerves, and abnormal auditory EPs in acoustic neuroma.

POTENTIAL FINDINGS

See above. It is important to realise that the nature of the underlying lesion is not evident from evoked potential results. Thus identical evoked potential results may follow from multiple sclerosis or a tumour on the optic nerve.

PATIENT ADVICE

- Electrodes will be placed on the skin or scalp, and the jelly that is used may necessitate hair-washing later.
- Patients must bring their glasses for visual evoked potential testing, which takes about 20 minutes.
- Brainstem testing takes about 40 minutes, and somatosensory tests, which are technically more difficult, take up to 60 minutes.

Other investigations

1 Lumbar puncture (LP)

DESCRIPTION

In adults the spinal cord ends at L2, and CSF may be sampled by inserting a needle under local anaesthetic through the supraspinous ligament and dura, into the subarachnoid space at L3–4, or occasionally L2–3 or L4–5. CSF pressure can be measured with a manometer attached to the lumbar-puncture needle before CSF is collected.

INDICATIONS AND POTENTIAL FINDINGS

- CSF abnormalities include infection (e.g. meningitis), blood (e.g. subarachnoid haemorrhage), cells and immunoglobulins (e.g. multiple sclerosis).

- Specific tests include particular viral antibodies (e.g. progressive multifocal leucoencephalopathy).
- CSF pressure may be elevated in benign intracranial hypertension.

RELATED INVESTIGATIONS

If LP fails even under X-ray control, lateral cervical puncture may be performed under X-ray control.

PATIENT ADVICE

- The test is performed under local anaesthetic on the bed, casualty trolley or X-ray table.
- The patient lies comfortably on his or her side with the back and legs flexed. Pillows may be used to prevent him or her from rolling forward.
- Lignocaine is injected into the skin and subcutaneous tissues so that the patient feels only pressure after the initial needle prick.
- CSF is allowed to drain (not aspirated), and CSF pressure measurement is standard practice, so a few minutes' wait after successful stylet insertion is normal, as is simultaneous blood glucose measurement.
- The patient will need to rest for a few hours, and may go home later that day.

GP ADVICE

- The most common complication is post-LP headache due to continued CSF leakage through the dural hole. Headache is worse on standing and sitting, and is relieved by bed rest. The great majority of people who develop post-LP headache do so within 48 hours, and most do so within 24 hours. Treatment is bed rest with paracetamol analgesia if necessary and adequate fluids. If headache is particularly prolonged, an epidural blood patch may be used in hospital.
- Other complications are rare. Prolonged or severe lumbar back pain, evidence of central nervous system infection, or signs of cord or root compression necessitate re-referral to the unit that performed the test. The most serious complications are transtentorial herniation or cerebellar tonsillar herniation (coning). This has not been reported in general practice for patients discharged following LP. It occurs when obstruction/leakage of CSF or a mass lesion in the head causes pressure differences between intracranial compartments and the vertebral canal, with consequent transtentorial herniation of the medial temporal lobes or tonsillar herniation (of cerebellar tonsils and medulla

through the foramen magnum). Any patient with a decreasing level of consciousness or who develops third-nerve palsy or any other neurological deficit after LP requires referral to a neurosurgery unit.

2 Muscle biopsy

DESCRIPTION

Biopsies are performed under local anaesthetic in limb muscles such as the vastus lateralis or deltoid. Closed biopsies are quick, day-case procedures that are performed on the ward. Open biopsies under local anaesthetic in theatre are preferable in some situations (e.g. severe atrophy).

INDICATIONS

- To determine whether muscle weakness is due to myopathy or dystrophy, or is neurogenic in origin.
- To screen for inborn errors of metabolism.

POTENTIAL FINDINGS

Histology, histochemistry and sometimes electron microscopy help to differentiate between the following:

- dystrophies – with abnormal muscle-fibre appearance, necrosis and replacement with fatty or fibrous tissue;
- myopathies – with necrosis, inflammatory cell infiltrate and fibrosis;
- neurogenic problems – atrophy of fibres supplied by a single motor unit.

PATIENT ADVICE

- The patient may be re-examined because the muscle biopsied should be moderately affected but not atrophied and end-stage.
- Muscles which have been sampled by EMG are avoided.
- More than one sample is frequently taken from a single incision, and more than one area may be sampled because changes can be patchy in distribution.
- Closed biopsies require only steristrips and a dry dressing. The limb should not be used vigorously for 24 hours and should be kept clean and dry for 72 hours after the procedure.

GP ADVICE

Open biopsies may require sutures and should be treated like a minor surgical incision.

3 Psychometric (or neuropsychometric) testing

DESCRIPTION

These are detailed tests performed by a clinical psychologist, either in pen-and-paper format or by computer.

INDICATIONS AND POTENTIAL FINDINGS

Investigation of cognitive or behavioural change, such as occurs in head injury or dementia. Many higher functions are tested, including verbal and visual memory, executive functions of planning and organisation, language, visuospatial abilities, constructional tasks, and current and estimated premorbid IQ. Screening tests for anxiety, depression and other psychological disorders may be included.

PATIENT ADVICE

Testing is prolonged and may be conducted in more than one session in order to reduce patient fatigue. Interviews about family background, early experiences, education and vocational history, and previous psychological or psychiatric contact are standard.

4 Tensilon test

DESCRIPTION

Edrophonium (Tensilon) is given intravenously to briefly prolong the action of acetylcholine at the neuromuscular junction.

INDICATIONS

To investigate possible myasthenia gravis.

POTENTIAL FINDINGS

- In a positive test the power of weak muscles improves, within 30–60 seconds of injection, for a few minutes. Bulbar and respiratory muscles can be tested by assessing speech and testing vital capacity.

- The test may be equivocal in polymyositis or motor neurone disease, and false-negative results may occur (e.g. in ocular myasthenia).

RELATED INVESTIGATIONS

Single-fibre EMG, nerve stimulation tests, blood tests for acetylcholine-receptor antibodies and CT of the mediastinum to check for thymoma or other tumours.

PATIENT ADVICE

The drug is given intravenously and may induce muscarinic side effects, including salivation, sweating and lacrimation. Intravenous access will be maintained during the test because bradycardia and hypotension can occur.

OBSTETRICS AND GYNAECOLOGY

Pelvic ultrasound

Diagnostic laparoscopy

Colposcopy

Hysteroscopy and endometrial sampling

Hysterosalpingogram (HSG)

Urodynamic investigations

Prenatal diagnosis

OBSTETRICS AND GYNAECOLOGY

Elizabeth S Payne

Pelvic ultrasound

DESCRIPTION

The introduction of ultrasound examination of the pelvis has revolutionised the practice of clinical gynaecology, and in many cases has eliminated the need for admission for invasive surgical diagnostic procedures.

Ultrasound examination of the female pelvis is probably the most valuable aid to the management of gynaecological problems. It is often available to GPs by direct access, although waiting times for non-urgent examination may be lengthy.

The pelvis may be visualised either abdominally via a full bladder or using a transvaginal approach. In many departments, both routes are utilised at each examination in order to obtain the maximum amount of information. The abdominal route is used in the assessment of a large pelvic mass and allows the visualisation of ascitic fluid and evidence of hydronephrosis or liver secondaries. In obese patients, it may be impossible to visualise the pelvic organs adequately, and the transvaginal approach may then be indicated.

Transvaginal scanning has the advantage of enabling the probe to be placed much closer to the structures to be inspected, and it also avoids the need for a full bladder. However, some patients are unhappy about the concept of the vaginal approach, and in young children, women who are virgo intacta or suffer from vaginismus, and in the elderly with very atrophic vaginas, this approach would be inappropriate.

INDICATIONS

- Investigation of a pelvic mass.
- Investigation of pelvic pain.
- Diagnosis of pregnancy and investigation of pain and/or bleeding in early pregnancy.
- Investigation of subfertility.

- Investigation of post-menopausal bleeding.
- Investigation of a 'lost' intrauterine contraceptive device.

POTENTIAL FINDINGS

- **Uterus**: size and position.

- **Fibroids**: if present, these may be visualised and their number, size, disposition, and evidence of calcification or degeneration may be reported. In the case of large pedunculated fibroids, it may not be possible to visualise their continuity with the uterus.

- **Endometrium**: the endometrial thickness is routinely measured. Excessive thickening or irregularity may be suggestive of hyperplasia, malignancy or endometrial polyps.

- **Fallopian tubes**: normal Fallopian tubes are not visualised. Tubal pathology including hydrosalpinx or pyosalpinx should be visible, but can be difficult to distinguish from loops of bowel. The patency of normal tubes can be assessed using a technique whereby fluid that can be ultrasonically visualised is instilled into the uterine cavity and can be seen as it passes along the tubes.

- **Ovaries**: these may be difficult to visualise, especially in post-menopausal women, and may be obscured by bowel. A change of position may overcome this problem. Ultrasound examination usually enables size, shape and presence of cysts to be visualised. Cysts will be described in terms of their size and nature (cystic or solid, simple or complex), and may be further assessed by Doppler for measurement of blood flow, which would be increased in malignancy. Ultrasound examination of the ovaries is also helpful in making the diagnosis of polycystic ovarian syndrome, in which the ovaries are typically enlarged with increased stroma and contain multiple small cysts (typically 5–8 mm in diameter) that are peripherally distributed.

- **Early pregnancy problems**: ultrasound examination is the most helpful tool in the assessment of pain and bleeding in early pregnancy. Using the transvaginal approach it may be possible to see an intrauterine sac from as early as 10 days following the first missed period. Sometimes it is not possible to state definitively at the first scan whether a pregnancy is viable, and a repeat scan 10 to 14 days later may be indicated. If ectopic pregnancy is suspected, an ultrasound scan may be helpful in confirming that the pregnancy is intrauterine, or may be suggestive of an ectopic pregnancy if thickened endometrium and an empty uterus in association with an adnexal mass is noted. However, it must be remembered that an ultrasound scan can never completely exclude an ectopic gestation – if clinical findings suggest this diagnosis, laparoscopy is the definitive investigation.

- **Subfertility**: ultrasound examination may aid the investigation in several ways, including assessment of ovarian morphology, determination of the size and number of developing follicles, serial follicle tracking for assessment of ovulation and assessment of endometrial thickness.

PATIENT ADVICE

- The patient is usually advised to attend with a full bladder.
- The procedure will be performed in a darkened ultrasound-examination room, and the pelvic structures or early pregnancy can be seen on the television monitor.
- For abdominal examination, the abdomen will need to be exposed from the costal margin to the symphysis pubis.
- The procedure is usually quite painless, but pressure on the full bladder may sometimes cause minor discomfort.
- For transvaginal examination, the patient is required to undress from the waist down and will be asked to lie in the same position as for any other vaginal examination, with the legs drawn up and the vulva exposed.
- The vaginal probe, which is covered by a clean, protective condom, is gently introduced within the vagina. Movement of the probe may result in some discomfort but rarely causes any significant pain.

GP ADVICE

Ultrasound examination reports must be interpreted in conjunction with the history and clinical findings. In many situations it may not be possible to give a definitive diagnosis (e.g. to distinguish between a fibroid and a solid ovarian cyst, or to confirm that a pregnancy is viable) or to recognise significant pathology (e.g. endometriosis or pelvic inflammatory disease).

Diagnostic laparoscopy

DESCRIPTION

Laparoscopy is a technique that allows direct inspection of the pelvis and intra-abdominal organs for evidence of pathology. It is generally performed under general anaesthetic and requires admission to hospital, usually as a day case.

INDICATIONS AND POTENTIAL FINDINGS

- Investigations of pelvic pain, secondary dysmenorrhoea or dyspareunia.
- Investigation of subfertility.
- Investigation of a possible pelvic mass, including ovarian cysts.
- For diagnosis of ectopic gestation.
- For assessment prior to either possible tubal surgery or consideration of reversal of sterilisation.
- For the initial diagnosis of endometriosis or to assess response to medical therapy.
- Rarely, to confirm the diagnosis of acute pelvic inflammatory disease and to obtain bacteriological samples.

Sometimes it may be possible to undertake simple surgical procedures at the time of diagnostic laparoscopy. Such procedures include the following:

- aspiration of simple ovarian cysts;
- division of adhesions;
- laser ablation or diathermy of endometrial deposits;
- management of an unruptured ectopic pregnancy;
- ovarian diathermy in the treatment of polycystic ovarian syndrome.

PATIENT ADVICE

- Diagnostic laparoscopy can usually be preformed as a day-case procedure and takes about 20 minutes.
- The patient will require a short general anaesthetic.
- The abdomen is first distended with carbon dioxide gas.
- A small incision is made just below the umbilicus and a laparoscope is inserted into the abdominal cavity. It may be necessary to make a second small incision in the lower abdomen to enable a pair of forceps to be inserted in order to manipulate the pelvic structures.
- On completion of the procedure the gas is released and the incision(s) closed with a single dissolvable suture.
- Diagnostic laparoscopy usually causes mild to moderate lower abdominal pain, and may also cause referred pain in the shoulders due to entrapment of gas beneath the diaphragm.

- Simple analgesia is usually adequate, and opiate analgesia is rarely required.
- Following laparoscopy, the patient should be escorted home by a responsible adult who should stay with her for at least 12 hours.
- The patient should be advised to rest and avoid strenuous activity for 48–72 hours after the procedure.

GP ADVICE

Post-operatively, the pain should not be severe and the abdomen should be soft with no rebound or guarding. If the patient complains of persistent severe pain with any evidence of peritonism or damage to an intra-abdominal organ, bleeding should be suspected and readmission arranged urgently.

Colposcopy

DESCRIPTION

Colposcopy allows direct visualisation of the cervix under low-power magnification, and is used in the assessment of abnormal cervical cytology or known or suspected cervical pathology. GPs can arrange referral directly to a specialist colposcopy clinic according to guidance given on the cervical cytology result forms.

INDICATIONS

- Two or more inadequate smears.
- Two or more inflammatory smears which have failed to return to normal after appropriate treatment of infection.
- Any smear showing dyskaryosis.
- Any smear showing potentially malignant cells.
- Any woman with a cervix that has a suspicious appearance, even if cytology is negative.

POTENTIAL FINDINGS AND PATIENT ADVICE

- Prior to referral for colposcopy for investigation of an abnormal smear the patient should be reassured that abnormal cervical cytology does not mean cervical cancer.

- Colposcopy is usually an out-patient procedure and takes about 20 minutes.
- The patient will be required to undress from the waist down, and to lie on an examination couch with her legs up in stirrups.
- The cervix will be exposed by means of a speculum and will be gently painted with diluted acetic acid and/or iodine solution before being inspected via the colposcope. This allows the presence and extent of any lesions to be determined accurately.
- Any abnormal areas may be biopsied. This may give rise to a brief 'pinching' sensation, but should not cause any significant pain or bleeding.
- It may be possible to reassure the patient that there is no significant pathology at the initial visit. She may then return to the routine cervical cytology screening programme. Alternatively, it may be necessary to await histological diagnosis on the basis of the biopsy result, which usually takes about 1 to 2 weeks.
- In certain circumstances, the patient may be advised that it would be appropriate to proceed directly to a loop cone biopsy of the cervix at the initial consultation.

Loop cone biopsy of the cervix

This is performed with local anaesthetic under direct colposcopic visualisation. Local anaesthetic is injected into each of the four quadrants of the ectocervix. When the anaesthetic has taken effect, a large biopsy is taken using a specially designed wire loop and cutting diathermy. This procedure takes about 5 minutes and is associated with minimal pain or bleeding. Following the procedure the patient will be advised to rest for a short time. She will also be advised to avoid the use of internal tampons and coitus for up to 6 weeks in order to facilitate healing.

GP ADVICE

The patient should be referred to the hospital if she has significant offensive discharge, fresh bleeding or severe pain.

Hysteroscopy and endometrial sampling

DESCRIPTION

Hysteroscopy is a technique that allows direct visualisation of the endometrium and the uterine cavity. This procedure was initially performed under general anaesthesia, but the development of smaller 5-mm endoscopes has enabled it to be undertaken as an out-patient procedure. Many hospitals now provide direct-access hysteroscopy clinics which allow 'one-stop' investigation for menstrual problems and post-menopausal bleeding. Hysteroscopically directed endometrial biopsy may be performed at the same time.

INDICATIONS

- Menorrhagia.
- Intermenstrual bleeding.
- Post-menopausal bleeding.
- Investigation of abnormal bleeding in association with use of hormone replacement therapy (HRT).

POTENTIAL FINDINGS

- Hysteroscopy allows the size and regularity of the uterine cavity to be assessed. It is possible to recognise submucous fibroids, fibroid polyps, endometrial polyps and intrauterine adhesions.
- The endometrium can also be inspected, and atrophic changes, endometrial hyperplasia or malignancy recognised and any abnormality biopsied under direct vision.

PATIENT ADVICE

- Hysteroscopy may be undertaken either as an out-patient procedure or as a day-case procedure under general anaesthesia.
- For an out-patient procedure, the patient will be required to undress from the waist down and to lie on an examination/colposcopy couch with her legs in stirrups.
- The cervix will be exposed using a speculum and, after cleansing the area, the hysteroscope is gently introduced through the cervical canal into the uterine cavity.

- The procedure usually causes no more than mild to moderate discomfort, but if the patient experiences significant discomfort or pain a paracervical block may be administered.

- On completion of the procedure, the patient may be advised to rest for a while and should then be accompanied home by a friend or relative.

GP ADVICE

Following the procedure, mild 'period-like' pain may occur for a few hours and should respond to simple analgesia. Occasionally there may also be slight spotting of blood which will settle spontaneously within 1 or 2 days.

Hysterosalpingogram (HSG)

DESCRIPTION

This is a test of tubal patency using a radio-opaque dye which is instilled via the uterus. It is usually available by direct access to GPs, and is generally performed during the course of investigations of subfertility.

INDICATIONS AND POTENTIAL FINDINGS

- Assessment of tubal patency/pathology during investigation of subfertility.

- Assessment of correct placement of clips and occlusion of tubes following tubal ligation/sterilisation procedures.

- Assessment of the uterine cavity for evidence of submucous fibroids or congenital uterine anomalies during the investigation of subfertility or recurrent miscarriage.

- Assessment of cervical incompetence in the investigation of recurrent miscarriage.

- To diagnose intrauterine adhesions in Aschermann's syndrome.

PATIENT ADVICE

The patient will be asked to telephone the X-ray department on the first day of her menstrual period in order to book an appointment for a hysterosalpingogram. HSG is usually performed within the first 10 days of the cycle in order to avoid the risk of exposing a very early pregnancy to radiation.

- The patient should be advised to attend on the day of the test with an adult friend or relative who will be able to accompany her home by car or taxi, as she may experience mild to severe 'period-like' pain that causes her to feel faint.

- The test is performed in a darkened X-ray room and takes about 20 minutes.

- The patient will be required to undress from the waist down and to lie on an examination table with her legs drawn up and the vulva exposed. The cervix is visualised using a speculum, and is gently cleansed prior to the introduction of a cannula into the cervical canal. The radio-opaque dye is then instilled into the uterus and will flow along the Fallopian tubes.

- If there is any evidence of tubal pathology, the patient will be given prophylactic antibiotics.

- Following the procedure simple analgesia should be adequate.

GP ADVICE

HSG is able to confirm tubal patency. This does not equate to normal tubal function. If tubal pathology is demonstrated, it is often necessary to proceed to diagnostic laparoscopy for further assessment of the external aspects of the tubes and the remainder of the pelvis in order to decide on the most appropriate management.

Urodynamic investigations

DESCRIPTION AND INDICATIONS

- Urodynamic investigations are now widely available in most gynaecological departments. They help to discriminate between genuine stress incontinence (GSI) and urgency and urge incontinence.

- Testing is usually performed in a specialist unit, by either a specially trained doctor or a specialist nurse.

- Catheters in the bladder and rectum allow for the continuous recording of both intra-vesical and intra-abdominal pressure.

POTENTIAL FINDINGS

Urodynamic testing allows a range of urological parameters to be assessed, including the following:

- maximum bladder capacity;
- bladder capacity at first urge to void;
- evidence of detrusor instability;
- urethral pressure;
- completeness of voiding;
- evidence of incontinent episodes.

Interpretation of the findings should provide a diagnosis (e.g. stable bladder with evidence of GSI, or unstable bladder with detrusor instability).

PATIENT ADVICE

- Urodynamic investigations are performed as an out-patient procedure and take 20–30 minutes to complete.
- The patient will be required to undress from the waist down prior to passage of the catheters.
- She should experience no more than mild discomfort during the procedure, and must be advised that episodes of incontinence are common.
- On completion of the procedure she may resume normal daily activities and should not require any analgesia.

GP ADVICE

Urodynamic studies are rarely available to GPs by direct referral. This is because the results require specialist interpretation and, unless a detailed report is provided, most GPs would experience great difficulty in interpreting the resultant pressure recordings.

Prenatal diagnosis

In recent years there have been several major advances in techniques available for prenatal diagnosis, including the development of chorionic villus sampling (CVS) in the first trimester, the use of DNA techniques for diagnosis of single-gene disorders and early amniocentesis (at 13 weeks). Whatever type of test is being considered, counselling is of paramount importance. Although trained counsellors are available in most antenatal clinics, the role of the GP who knows the patient, her family and personal circumstances cannot be underestimated.

TESTS USED IN PRENATAL DIAGNOSIS

- Chromosomal analysis for the following:
  family history of chromosomal abnormality; pregnancies shown to be at higher risk for a chromosomal anomaly as a result of prenatal serum screening tests; maternal age over 35 years.

- DNA analysis for single-gene disorders, usually based on family history of a previously affected child.

- Biochemical analysis for certain metabolic disorders.

Most prenatal diagnostic tests can be performed using either tissue obtained at CVS or fluid obtained at amniocentesis. However, for some metabolic disorders and subtle chromosome abnormalities, tests can only be performed on samples obtained at amniocentesis.

1 Chorionic villus sampling

DESCRIPTION

This procedure involves sampling of placental tissue, and has the advantage that it can be performed during the first trimester. As results are usually available within 3 to 4 days, in the event of an anomaly being confirmed, it is possible for the patient to undergo a first-trimester suction termination of pregnancy under general anaesthetic, which most women find very much less distressing. CVS is performed at about 11 weeks' gestation and is normally only undertaken in regional and subregional centres.

PATIENT ADVICE

- This is an out-patient procedure, it takes about 20 minutes and the usual route is transabdominal.

- It is performed in the ultrasound department, and the patient will be required to lie on a scan couch with her lower abdomen exposed.

- An ultrasound scan is performed to check the fetus and to locate the position of the placenta.

- A local anaesthetic is injected into the skin of the patient's abdomen, and under ultrasound guidance a fine needle is passed through the abdomen and into the placenta. Tissue from the placenta is then gently aspirated.

- Occasionally it is necessary to repeat the procedure once more in order to obtain a larger sample.

- Following the procedure, the needle is withdrawn and a further ultrasound examination is performed in order to confirm that the fetus is alive and unharmed.

- The patient should be accompanied home by a responsible adult friend or relative, and should rest for the remainder of the day.

- Most women describe the test as uncomfortable rather than painful.

GP ADVICE

Some women experience low abdominal pain or slight vaginal bleeding, which should settle within 1 or 2 days. Chromosome results are usually available within 2 to 10 days. DNA analysis or biochemical testing may take a little longer. The miscarriage rate following CVS is estimated to be between 1 in 50 and 1 in 100 cases. The slightly higher risk of miscarriage with CVS is offset by the advantage of avoiding a second-trimester termination. Rarely, due to placental mosaicism, it may not be possible to obtain a definitive result. In these circumstances, it is still possible to have amniocentesis performed at 16 weeks' gestation, such that a result can still be obtained.

2 Amniocentesis

DESCRIPTION

This procedure involves aspiration of amniotic fluid, and can usually be performed in the patient's local obstetric unit unless very specialised biochemical testing is required. It is usually undertaken at 16–18 weeks, and the results are available within 2 to 3 weeks. Consequently, by the time they are available, the pregnancy is already well advanced into the second trimester, the mother will have felt fetal movements and, if an abnormality is confirmed, will be in the sad position of having to contemplate a second-trimester termination of pregnancy.

PATIENT ADVICE

- Amniocentesis is also an out-patient procedure which takes 5–10 minutes.

- It is performed under ultrasound control in the scan department.

- The patient will be asked to lie down on a scan couch with her lower abdomen exposed.

- Following an ultrasound scan to determine the position of the fetus and the placenta, and to identify the largest pools of liquor, a local anaesthetic will be injected into the skin. A fine needle is then passed gently through the abdominal wall into the fluid around the fetus and about 10 mL of fluid are drawn off.

- The needle is removed and a further scan is performed to check the fetus.
- The procedure is slightly uncomfortable, but it is not painful.
- The woman should be accompanied to the test and should avoid driving home. She should then rest for the remainder of the day.
- The miscarriage rate following amniocentesis is estimated to be between 1 in 100 and 1 in 150 cases.

GP ADVICE

Although most pregnancy losses following amniocentesis occur within 2 to 3 weeks of the procedure due to either rupture of the membranes or the development of intrauterine infection, later losses due to pre-term labour and delivery may occur.

OPHTHALMOLOGY

Visual-field testing

Tonometry

Fluorescein angiography

Keratometry

A-ultrasound

Orthoptic assessment

Radiological investigations

B-ultrasound

Electrophysiology

OPHTHALMOLOGY

Hunter Maclean

Most investigations in ophthalmology are more or less painless and non-invasive. Generally, GPs have little scope for direct access to these investigations, as most of them require either specialist skills in performing the investigation or specialist experience in interpreting the results. However, it is increasingly common to find GPs working in ophthalmic clinics, and some of them have transferred skills gained here to the GP surgery, although this often involves the purchase of expensive equipment. Ophthalmic opticians are using increasingly sophisticated equipment, and many boast automated visual-field analysers, slit lamps and tonometry (measurement of intra-ocular pressure). Thus appropriate referral to an optician can sometimes be helpful.

Some of these investigations are relatively rare but they do crop up in letters to GPs, and so the following account may help to make sense of what is happening to their patients.

Visual-field testing

DESCRIPTION

There are many ways of measuring visual fields, ranging from simple confrontation assessment to fully automated visual-field analysers. The latter are generally used in ophthalmic departments and by opticians.

INDICATIONS

- Assessment of glaucomatous damage.
- Assessment of neurological field defects (e.g. hemianopias).
- Assessment of ability to drive a car.

POTENTIAL FINDINGS

A major finding is the extent of a patient's central 30 degrees of visual field. The Driver and Vehicle Licensing Agency (DVLA) stipulates a minimum visual field required for a person to hold a driving licence. This is an uninterrupted area of vision 60 degrees wide either side of fixation (a total of 120 degrees) and 40 degrees tall. The test is carried out with both eyes open.

RELATED INVESTIGATIONS

- Used in conjunction with tonometry and optic-disc assessment, visual-field examination forms one of the cornerstones of glaucoma diagnosis and follow-up.

- Discovery of a neurological visual-field defect such as a bitemporal hemianopia will lead to further radiological studies such as MRI or CT scanning.

PATIENT ADVICE

- The patient is seated in front of an illuminated bowl and one eye is patched.

- The patient is asked to maintain central fixation while the machine projects spots of light into the bowl. If these are seen, the patient responds by pressing a button. Normally only the central 30 degrees of visual field are measured, as this is where most pathology is found.

- The test duration can vary from 3 to 20 minutes per eye depending on the sophistication of the programme.

- There is a learning curve, but even so some patients are unable to produce meaningful results with this test. Patients often erroneously feel that they are performing badly in these tests and so start to guess, thus making the test findings uninterpretable. It is important to reassure the patient that there is a learning curve and that allowances are made for patient errors during the test.

GP ADVICE

- The extent of a normal visual field in one eye is governed by facial characteristics such as the size of a person's nose or the overhang of their brow. On average, one eye will have a visual field 150 degrees wide and 120 degrees tall. Thus having only one functioning eye is not a bar to holding a driving licence.

- Laser treatment for proliferative diabetic retinopathy can lead to loss of a driving licence through destruction of visual field. All patients undergoing such treatment must be warned of this possibility.

Tonometry

DESCRIPTION

Goldmann tonometry involves instilling local anaesthetic and fluorescein drops into the conjunctival sac. The intra-ocular pressure is measured using a tonometer mounted on a slit lamp, which is brought into contact with the cornea. Other methods exist, including non-contact tonometry, which use a puff of air. These methods are popular with opticians but are not always accurate.

INDICATIONS

- Measurement of intra-ocular pressure.
- Assessment of glaucoma.

POTENTIAL FINDINGS

- High intra-ocular pressure.
- Low intra-ocular pressure.

RELATED INVESTIGATIONS

Used in conjunction with visual-field examination and optic-disc assessment, tonometry forms one of the cornerstones of glaucoma diagnosis and follow-up.

PATIENT ADVICE

- This is a painless procedure apart from the fact that, after instillation, the anaesthetic drops sting for about 10 seconds.

GP ADVICE

It is not uncommon for GPs to receive letters from opticians reporting high intra-ocular pressures in a particular patient. Many of these readings turn out to be false-positives, but nonetheless these patients require referral for further assessment. If the intra-ocular pressure is genuinely raised, then a diagnosis of glaucoma is made if there is coexisting optic nerve/visual field damage, or of ocular hypertension if no damage is found.

Fluorescein angiography

DESCRIPTION

Fluorescein dye (3–5 mL) is injected into a peripheral vein (in some centres under certain circumstances indocyanine green dye is used instead). After about 20 seconds the dye can be seen and photographed in the retinal circulation. Serial photographs are taken over the first few minutes, and are sometimes followed by late photographs approximately 20 minutes later.

INDICATIONS

- Investigation of diabetic retinopathy.
- Investigation of macular degeneration/other macular lesions.
- Diagnosis/quantification of retinal ischaemia.
- Diagnosis of papilloedema.
- Diagnosis of new vessels.

POTENTIAL FINDINGS

- Leakage of fluorescein dye from the retinal circulation is abnormal, as the retinal circulation is an extension of the blood–brain barrier. The pattern of leakage can often be helpful in the diagnosis of certain conditions, such as macular lesions. New vessels leak fluorescein profusely and are usually obvious to the experienced observer.
- Dark patches which show no dye are non-perfused areas and so are diagnostic of retinal ischaemia.
- In some cases early papilloedema can be difficult to diagnose on fundoscopy, and in these situations fluorescein angiography is often helpful.

RELATED INVESTIGATIONS

Fluorescein angiography is not a substitute for a thorough fundal examination. In many cases, an examination of the fundus precludes the need for fluorescein angiography.

PATIENT ADVICE

- Fluorescein can cause transient nausea and discoloration of the skin and urine of some patients reminiscent of jaundice.
- The patient should be aware that in many cases an angiogram is being performed with future laser treatment in mind. In some centres this will occur on the same day.

GP ADVICE

Fluorescein angiograms are most commonly carried out to investigate macular degeneration and diabetic retinopathy.

Keratometry

DESCRIPTION

This procedure consists of a measurement of the corneal curvature in two axes 90 degrees apart.

INDICATIONS

- Assessment of astigmatism.
- Calculation of intra-ocular lens power (see section below on 'Related investigations').

POTENTIAL FINDINGS

If the corneal curvature is the same in each axis, then the cornea is a perfect dome shape. However, if there is a difference between the axes then astigmatism is said to be present. The steeper the curve of the lens, the more powerful it becomes. Thus corneas are of varying power depending on the steepness of their curvature. This is important when choosing the power of an intra-ocular lens to be implanted during cataract surgery.

RELATED INVESTIGATIONS

Together with A-ultrasound (see below) to measure axial length, keratometry forms the basis for calculation of the intra-ocular lens power (biometry) to be used after cataract extraction.

PATIENT ADVICE

The patient puts his or her chin on a rest in a similar fashion to a slit lamp and an optical measurement is taken from the cornea. No contact is involved.

GP ADVICE

See A-ultrasound below.

A-ultrasound

DESCRIPTION

This procedure involves ultrasonic measurement of the axial length of the eye.

INDICATION

This procedure represents one part of biometry (see above).

POTENTIAL FINDINGS

An accurate measurement of the length of the eye.

RELATED INVESTIGATIONS

Calculation of the intra-ocular lens power (biometry).

PATIENT ADVICE

- After the cornea has been anaesthetised with drops, an ultrasound probe is placed on the cornea and measurements of the axial length of the eye are taken.
- This is a painless procedure but it does require the patient to keep the eye still during examination.
- Biometry is usually performed in hospital about 2 weeks before operation. At this time the procedure for the cataract surgery is explained in detail.

GP ADVICE

- Occasionally, readings cannot be taken because of poor patient co-operation or the presence of such a dense cataract that the ultrasound wave does not penetrate the eye.

- Although biometry is accurate in the majority of cases, inaccuracies do occur in patients who have very long or short eyes. Surprises do occasionally occur, and can be managed either optically or by exchanging the implant in a further operation.

Orthoptic assessment

DESCRIPTION

Orthoptics is the study of the balance between the eyes.

INDICATIONS

Orthoptists are paramedical technicians who are experts in the detection, measurement and follow-up of squints, assessment of double vision and measurement of vision in children.

POTENTIAL FINDINGS

- In children, orthoptic examination detects and characterises amblyopia, squint and other disorders of eye balance (e.g. nystagmus).
- For adults, onset of a squint leads to double vision, and assessment of this by an orthoptist can differentiate between various cranial nerve palsies, thyroid eye disease and various myopathies such as myasthenia gravis.

RELATED INVESTIGATIONS

Full neurological examination and ophthalmic examination.

PATIENT ADVICE

- A variety of optical tests are used. They are painless and generally require only the co-operation of the patient.
- Children with suspected squints or other problems will usually be seen by both an ophthalmologist and an orthoptist.

GP ADVICE

After an initial assessment of children with squint, follow-up visits are often with the orthoptist alone, who monitors the child's response to treatments such as patching. If there is treatment failure, or surgery for a squint is thought to be appropriate, then the patient will be redirected to the ophthalmologist.

Radiological investigations

INDICATIONS AND POTENTIAL FINDINGS

Standard X-rays, CT scanning and MRI scanning are performed in the usual way, and the latter are frequently used to investigate unexplained visual failure or proptosis. Ultrasound Duplex scanning and angiography are used to investigate the carotid arteries. Plain X-rays are not much used in ophthalmology, except for excluding blow-out fractures of the inferior orbit in a casualty setting. CT scanning and MRI scanning are used to investigate masses in the orbit and pituitary fossa. Typically these include meningiomas, gliomas, lymphomas, haemangiomas and pituitary tumours. Swollen muscle bellies that are so typical of thyroid eye disease can also be demonstrated. Duplex scanning is useful in the investigation of amaurosis fugax, as it can demonstrate stenosis of the carotid arteries, which may require carotid endarterectomy.

PATIENT ADVICE

In the case of MRI scanning, it is important to make sure that the patient is not carrying any metal, including aneurysm clips, pacemakers and artificial joints.

GP ADVICE

Young patients or patients with claustrophobia may be difficult, if not impossible, to scan without a general anaesthetic.

B-ultrasound

DESCRIPTION

This procedure involves an ultrasonic examination of the intra-ocular contents and the orbit.

INDICATIONS AND POTENTIAL FINDINGS

- Commonly, B-ultrasound is used to detect retinal detachment when the ocular media are not clear (e.g. after a vitreous haemorrhage or in the presence of a dense cataract).

- It is also useful in the differential diagnosis and measurement of malignant melanoma, as these tumours have a characteristic ultrasound shadow.

- Examination of the extra-ocular muscles is also possible, and this can be helpful in the differential diagnosis of proptosis.

RELATED INVESTIGATIONS

Other radiological investigations, such as CT scanning and MRI scanning (see earlier).

PATIENT ADVICE

- The cornea is usually anaesthetised with drops and an ultrasound probe is placed on the eye, although a reasonable picture can be obtained by placing the probe on top of the closed lids.

- This is a painless procedure.

GP ADVICE

Patients – and especially diabetics with vitreous haemorrhages – may have regular ultrasound examinations to check the integrity of the retina while waiting for the blood to clear.

Electrophysiology

DESCRIPTION

Three separate tests can be performed, namely electroretinography, electro-oculography and visual evoked potentials. Each involves placing electrodes in contact with the eye or cranium, from which action potentials can be measured.

INDICATIONS AND POTENTIAL FINDINGS

Measurements are helpful in the diagnosis of demyelination of the optic nerve, and are particularly useful in the assessment of visual potential in infants and patients suspected of malingering.

RELATED INVESTIGATIONS

Further neurological and orthoptic assessment and examination.

PATIENT ADVICE

- The procedure is painless apart from the transitory effects of topical local anaesthesia.
- The eyes are stimulated either by flashes of light or by chequerboard patterns.

GP ADVICE

These tests are usually performed on infants who appear to be blind but are too young to be tested in the normal way.

ORTHOPAEDICS

Arthroscopy of the knee

Magnetic resonance imaging (MRI)

Isotope bone scanning

ORTHOPAEDICS

Richard Rawlins

Arthroscopy of the knee

DESCRIPTION

Arthrosopy involves endoscopic examination of a joint, and is usually a day-case procedure performed under a general anaesthetic. It can be conducted under local anaesthesia, but a general anaesthetic is usually preferred. Knee arthroscopy is preceded by an examination under anaesthetic, which gives useful information about cruciate and collateral ligaments.

The arthrosope, which is 4 mm wide, is inserted through various 'portals' along the joint line. An anterolateral stab incision beside the patella tendon will usually suffice. Examination probes can be placed through other portals and used to manipulate menisci, the cruciate ligaments, fat pads and plicae (synovial folds), and they can assess the firmness of articular cartilage.

The portals are closed with a small suture (which can be removed a week later) or simple sticking plaster.

INDICATIONS

- Knee pain.
- Functional disability, including locking, swelling, giving way, and inability to walk and/or run.

POTENTIAL FINDINGS

- This investigation helps to provide useful diagnostic and prognostic information, particularly for articular cartilage lesions. Key points include the presence of damage to the articular surface, the degree of damage and the compartments affected.
- It also helps to assess whether or not the patient is likely to benefit from a total knee replacement (lavage and debridement of articular cartilage may mitigate symptoms, at least for a while).

- If meniscal lesions are found, they can be operated on by repair, or by partial or total removal. Here the investigation enters therapeutic territory.
- If a cruciate ligament injury is identified, arthroscopy provides a clearer understanding of the full extent of the injury, any associated injury to menisci (which can be treated) and the decision as to whether reconstruction should be considered.

RELATED INVESTIGATIONS

CT and MRI have now largely superseded arthrograms. These tests are excellent for tears of menisci, although stability cannot be easily assessed. They are also useful for assessing cruciates, but are less helpful for assessing articular cartilage and do not provide an opportunity for therapy. CT or MRI can help to prioritise patients on a lengthy waiting-list for arthroscopy – if MRI shows a torn meniscus, a good case can be made for expediting treatment in case further damage is caused.

PATIENT ADVICE

- Risks are minimal.
- No pre-test preparation is required except for the anaesthetic.
- Post-test – early weight-bearing (usually immediately after the patient has recovered from the anaesthetic), and crutches until the patient is confident.
- Patients should have an information sheet provided by the surgeon detailing his or her advice with regard to post-operative care. Quadriceps exercises twice a day are advised until the patient is seen for review.
- Arthroscopy of the knee is a day-case procedure.

GP ADVICE

- Pain is rarely a problem. Treat with rest, elevation and non-steroidal anti-inflammatory drugs (NSAIDs).
- Infection is very rare, and when it does occur is usually only superficial, in the wounds. Minor local inflammation around the portals is common and should settle within a day or so.
- There is a theoretical possibility of septic arthritis, in which case the patient should be referred to hospital urgently. Suggestive symptoms include significant pain, swelling and pyrexia developing within 24–72 hours of the procedure. If in doubt, refer for urgent assessment.

Magnetic resonance imaging (MRI)

DESCRIPTION

Patients undergo this investigation on a table that is gradually inserted through the hole in the 'doughnut' shape of a large magnet. Computerised analysis of radio-wave deformation by different elements of body tissue provides a series of images similar to tomograms (MRI of course uses radio waves, not ionising radiation).

INDICATIONS AND POTENTIAL FINDINGS

Orthopaedic surgeons find MRI of most use in clarifying the complexity of intra-articular fractures and the relationship of tumours to vital structures, and in some cases in pre-operative planning for spinal surgery. It is rarely used as a primary investigation – standard radiograph images provide adequate information for the vast majority of straightforward diagnoses.

RELATED INVESTIGATIONS

- The results can only be assessed properly in conjunction with the appropriate radiographic film.
- Cervical computerised tomography is a newer development which has reduced the time taken for conventional CT from around 30 minutes to around 1 minute. Although in many cases CT has been superseded by MRI, the former does provide helpful information when dealing with fractures.

PATIENT ADVICE

- The procedure takes approximately 30 minutes, during which time some patients may experience claustrophobia.
- It is also very noisy, and has been likened by some to the sound of a pneumatic drill. Nevertheless, 95% of patients find the procedure entirely acceptable.
- It is possible to perform MRI on anaesthetised patients, but this is only necessary in exceptional cases.
- Patients' enthusiasm about 'having a scan' should be tempered by an under-standing of what the scan is designed to achieve (usually to help to plan a surgical procedure).

GP ADVICE

- Most imaging departments require GPs to refer patients through consultants, and direct access to MRI can usually only be arranged following an explanatory telephone call at least.

- MRI does require significant precautions if the patient has any inserted metallic implants. For this reason, a clear indication should be given to the radiologist as to whether the patient has undergone surgery (particularly neurosurgery).

- Pacemakers are a contraindication to MRI. In other respects no special preparation is required, and post-investigation adverse effects are highly unlikely.

Isotope bone scanning

DESCRIPTION

This investigation almost always involves injection of technetium (other isotopes are used sometimes). The scan itself takes place about 3 hours after the injection, by which time the technetium will have been incorporated into active bony sites. The scan takes place under a gamma camera not unlike an X-ray machine.

INDICATIONS

- The main indication is bone pain of unidentified cause, particularly if bone cancer (usually secondaries) is suspected.

- Orthopaedic surgeons may find a bone scan useful when investigating painful total joint replacements, to determine whether these are due to infection or loosening.

POTENTIAL FINDINGS

Scanning is non-specific and has to be carefully interpreted with reference to plain radiographs. In the case of secondary cancer, approximately 50% of the bony volume needs to be affected by tumour before radiographs will demonstrate the abnormality. Bone scanning may detect the disease when only 10% of the bony volume is affected.

RELATED INVESTIGATIONS

Bone scanning can only be properly assessed in conjunction with appropriate radiographic films.

PATIENT ADVICE

- This investigation is entirely risk free and takes approximately 45 minutes.
- The patient will have to attend 3 hours earlier for the injection, and in the intervening period they will be encouraged to drink as much as possible.

GP ADVICE

Bone scanning will normally only follow routine radiography, and for this reason is not an investigation which would generally be available to a GP without prior discussion with the radiologist.

OSTEOPOROSIS

Dual-energy X-ray absorptiometry (DXA)

OSTEOPOROSIS

Stuart Wood

Dual-energy X-ray absorptiometry (DXA)

DESCRIPTION

Although skeletal X-rays may provide a pointer to the existence of osteoporosis (e.g. wedge-compression fracture of lumbar vertebrae), it is necessary to measure bone density in order to make an accurate diagnosis. Several different methods exist, but the use of dual-energy X-ray absorptiometry (DXA) has emerged as the most acceptable technique in terms of reproducibility and its ability to measure bone mass at both axial and appendicular sites. Very low doses of radiation are used.

DXA bone scans are performed using a scanner which is substantial in both physical size and cost, and so is only likely to be available in specialist units in hospitals. For the patient, this means travelling, inconvenience and financial cost. As a result, there is some interest in other methods of measuring bone density, which are portable and can be used at the GP's surgery. Examples include a heel scanner, which also utilises DXA, and an ultrasound scanner, which is regarded more as an initial screening tool than as a reliable definitive measurement of bone mineral density (BMD).

INDICATIONS

- To confirm a clinical suspicion of osteoporosis (e.g. low-trauma fractures, spinal deformity, height loss, suggestive X-ray).

- To diagnose osteoporosis in those thought to be at risk:
    - (i) early menopause (< age 45 years) (*note that DXA is only indicated if it affects management – the patient is likely to be put on HRT in this situation in any case*);
    - (ii) significant episodes of amenorrhoea (> 6 months);
    - (iii) prolonged corticosteroid therapy (prednisolone > 7.5 mg daily for 6 months or longer);
    - (iv) primary hypogonadism;
    - (v) malabsorption;

(vi)   primary hyperparathyroidism;
(vii) chronic renal failure;
(viii) prolonged immobilisation;
(ix)   hyperthyroidism;
(x)   family history (this may be difficult to establish in practice);
(xi)   post-transplantation;
(xii) Cushing's syndrome.

- DXA also gives some quantitative measure of the severity of osteoporosis, and may have an increasing role in the monitoring of response to treatments intended to increase BMD.

POTENTIAL FINDINGS

The results of the BMD measurement obtained by DXA scan are absolute BMD, t-scores and z-scores (these are the number of standard deviations that the patient's result lies below the young adult average and the age-matched average, respectively). These results will usually be interpreted by the physician in charge of the DXA service, whether accessed directly or via a clinic. A t-score that is 2.5 standard deviations or more below the mean meets the World Health Organization (WHO) definition of osteoporosis (t-scores between -1 and -2.5 would qualify for a diagnosis of osteopenia).

RELATED INVESTIGATIONS

- X-ray examination has already been mentioned in association with osteoporosis. Its main use is in the diagnosis of fractures (including vertebral fractures). X-rays may also give a subjective impression of reduced BMD, but cannot be relied upon to diagnose or exclude osteoporosis.
- Ultrasound may be used as an initial screening tool (see above).
- Blood and urine tests to exclude other problems (e.g. osteomalacia or myeloma).

PATIENT ADVICE

- The patient can be reassured that a DXA bone scan is similar to having a skeletal X-ray, although the dose of radiation is very low.
- Whichever method is used, discomfort is minimal, and the patient is only required to lie still on the couch, sometimes with the knee flexed in the case of hip scans. Heel scans may involve the patient placing one heel in a water bath.

GP ADVICE

- This is not a particularly expensive test (approximate cost is £45).

- DXA normally gives fairly unambiguous results on which the doctor can base management decisions.

- There is scope for a significant increase in the number of patients for whom this scan would be appropriate – starting, for example, with those women who suffer a low-trauma wrist fracture.

PAEDIATRICS

Investigations for childhood urinary tract infections (UTIs)

Ultrasound for developmental dysplasia of the hips (DDH)

Sweat test

Small-intestinal biopsy

PAEDIATRICS

Vin Diwakar and Deirdre Kelly

The adage 'Children are not small adults' may sound trite, but must be considered when performing any investigation on a child. Anatomy and physiology change with age, and this is important when interpreting results. Four investigations which are more commonly performed in paediatric practice have been selected for discussion in this chapter.

Investigations for childhood urinary tract infections (UTIs)

BACKGROUND

Urinary tract infections (UTIs) are one of the commonest serious bacterial infections in infants and young children, with a reported prevalence of between 4.1% and 7.5%. Two primary aims guide the investigation of such children:

- the identification of anatomical abnormalities that predispose to infection;
- the prevention of renal scarring and its progression.

Most renal scars are present at diagnosis; it is unusual to develop them during follow-up. Thus scarring probably occurs during infancy, when the kidneys are maturing. This is when diagnosis of UTI is most difficult, as symptoms may be non-specific (e.g. poor feeding, lethargy and abdominal pain).

Although it is vital that the diagnosis of UTI is not missed in young infants, it is also essential that the diagnosis is accurate, in order that young children are not subjected to unnecessary, distressing and invasive procedures.

All urine specimens for bacteriology must be obtained after the perineum has been cleansed with soap and water. Antiseptic washes should be avoided, as they interfere with bacteriological growth. Co-operative children can provide a mid-stream specimen, but in infants and young children bag collection is used. The bag must be checked regularly and removed as soon as the specimen is produced in order to avoid contamination by skin commensals. If bag collection proves unsatisfactory, the infant may need a referral for suprapubic aspiration of urine or one-pass bladder catheterisation.

TYPES OF IMAGING AND INDICATIONS

Imaging modalities used in the initial investigation of UTI in children include the following:

- ultrasound;

- micturating cystourethrogram (MCUG);

- technetium-labelled dimercaptosuccinic acid renogram (DMSA).

All children of any age (variably defined as under the age of 12 to 16 years) with UTI require ultrasound examination of the urinary tract. This will show significant scarring and hence guide follow-up (e.g. further investigation, blood-pressure monitoring and repeat scans). Siblings of children with vesico-ureteric reflux require ultrasonography, as 30% of them will have the condition as well.

The exact ages at which other tests are indicated varies according to local radiological equipment and skills. The principle is that scarring is more likely to occur in infants aged less than 1 year. Children with unscarred kidneys at 3–4 years of age have a negligible risk of developing scars subsequently. Thus the investigation of the urinary tract is influenced by the child's age. GPs should be aware of this and should be involved in setting local policies.

DESCRIPTION AND POTENTIAL FINDINGS

- **Ultrasound:** anatomical abnormalities of the urinary tract, renal calculi and gross scars can be demonstrated, but small scars may be missed.

- **MCUG:** a urethral catheter is inserted to inject contrast into the bladder. The catheter is removed and the child is encouraged to void urine under screening. Important anatomical abnormalities of the bladder can be visualised, such as urethral valves in boys and ureterocoeles in girls, which both require surgery. Vesico-ureteric reflux can be demonstrated and graded.

- **DMSA scan:** intravenously injected radioactive isotope is taken up by renal tubules and retained. It demonstrates renal parenchyma damage, as scars do not take it up and appear as cold areas. An estimate of relative renal function can be made.

RELATED INVESTIGATIONS

MAG3 scan: technetium mercaptoacetyl triglycerine (MAG3) is filtered and excreted by the renal tubule. Renal perfusion and function can be quantified. When a diuretic is given, obstruction can be distinguished from non-obstuctive dilatation of the renal tract. The appearance of the tracer in the bladder and ureter during micturition can indirectly demonstrate vesico-ureteric reflux.

PATIENT ADVICE

- **Ultrasound:** some of the child's clothes will need to be removed for the scan, which takes 20–30 minutes. The child needs to be given plenty to drink before the scan, and if they are old enough, not allowed to pass urine for 1 hour before the scan.

- **MCUG:** the catheter is inserted and taped to the skin before the procedure. The radiologist then connects the catheter to a bottle of contrast, which looks just like water. Parents can watch the dye filling the bladder on the television screen. When the bladder is full, the child needs to micturate while they are still lying down on the table and X-rays are being taken. The entire procedure lasts 1–2 hours.

- **DMSA scan:** young children usually have local anaesthetic cream applied before venepuncture. The child lies on a bed, the isotope is injected and scans are taken for about 30 minutes. The child does not need to undress, and the parents may stay with the child. Children should have had something to drink within 60 minutes of the test. The radiation dose is less than that of an X-ray.

Ultrasound for developmental dysplasia of the hips (DDH)

DESCRIPTION

This test has two components.

- The depth and shape of the acetabulum are assessed by placing the ultrasound probe over the lateral aspect of the hip.

- Joint stability is evaluated by imaging the acetabulum and femoral head while performing a Barlow (flexion abduction) manoeuvre.

INDICATIONS

Ultrasound, usually at 4–6 weeks of age, is indicated in two groups:

- Infants with a hip 'click' or equivocal examination;

- Infants at high risk of DDH (i.e. family history of DDH, oligohydramnios, breech delivery, torticollis and foot deformity).

Ultrasound is most useful in infancy, as most of the hip joint is cartilaginous.

Some have argued for universal screening for DDH by ultrasound instead of physical examination. Such a programme would detect the small numbers of children with clinically silent DDH (abnormal ultrasound and normal physical examination), but may not be cost-effective and could lead to over-treatment.

RELATED INVESTIGATIONS

After 1 year, ossification of the femoral head means that ultrasound is no longer useful and plain radiography becomes more valuable.

PATIENT ADVICE

Portable ultrasound scanners enable scans to be undertaken in the paediatric or orthopaedic clinic by appropriately trained personnel, providing an immediate answer for parents.

GP ADVICE

The continuing debate over universal vs. targeted ultrasound screening means that GPs should be aware of and involved in setting local policy.

Sweat test

DESCRIPTION

The sweat test involves a quantitative analysis of sweat to determine electrolyte concentration, conductivity or osmolality. The test has three components:

- pilocarpine iontophoresis, in which a low-level electric current is applied to the test area, which may be on the arm or the leg, and must be free from rashes or inflammation. The positive electrode is covered with gauze and saturated with pilocarpine (which stimulates sweating). The negative electrode is covered with gauze and saturated with bicarbonate solution. The patient may experience a tingling sensation in the area, or a feeling of warmth. This part of the procedure takes approximately 5 minutes;
- 15–20 minutes after iontophoresis, the stimulated area is cleaned and the sweat collected on to gauze, filter paper, coil, patch or capillary tube;

- analysis of the sweat.

The entire procedure takes approximately 1 hour. At least 100 mg of sweat should be collected to ensure that there has been an adequate sweat rate, and infants should be at least 48 hours old before testing, because sweat electrolytes may be transiently elevated during the first 24 hours after birth.

INDICATIONS

- Recurrent respiratory disease or failure to thrive.
- Neonatal meconium ileus.
- A family history of cystic fibrosis (in a first-degree relative) or a positive newborn screen (performed in some areas).

POTENTIAL FINDINGS

- In children, the finding of a sweat sodium concentration greater than 60 mmol/L and sweat chloride concentration greater than 70 mmol/L is consistent with the diagnosis of cystic fibrosis (CF). Measurement of both sweat sodium and chloride is essential, as measurement of sweat sodium alone can be misleading. A positive test should always be confirmed at least once, since a range of conditions (including eczema) can give false-positive results.
- A sweat sodium concentration in the range 40–60 mmol/L is borderline and always warrants repetition of the test.
- A negative test should be repeated if the clinical picture is suggestive of CF.

RELATED INVESTIGATIONS

Some patients do present with a history suggestive of CF and persistently negative or borderline sweat test results. In such cases, mutation analysis can aid diagnosis. Mutation analysis is also used for carrier screening, prenatal diagnosis and newborn screening.

PATIENT ADVICE

- There are no restrictions on activity or diet or special preparations required before the test. However, creams or lotion should not be applied to the skin for 24 hours before the test. All regular medications may be continued.
- The result of the sweat test is usually made available on the next working day after the test is performed.

- In a small number of cases, the quantity of sweat obtained is not sufficient to give an accurate result, and the test may need to be repeated.

GP ADVICE

- Although we live in the age of molecular biology, the diagnosis of CF is still dependent on the sweat test, provided that it is performed by trained technicians who undertake sweat collection regularly, and that it is evaluated in a laboratory with experienced, reliable staff. The large number of mutations of the CF gene limits confirmation of the diagnosis by genetic analysis alone.
- There is a very small risk of a localised burn or urticaria at the site of the test.
- It is good practice to inform families of the result of a sweat test as soon as it is received.

Small-intestinal biopsy

DESCRIPTION

Two techniques are available, namely suction capsule biopsy and endoscopic biopsy. With both techniques, jejunal fluid is usually aspirated for microscopy and culture.

- **Suction biopsy:** this utilises a biopsy capsule containing a spring-loaded knife block that is attached to fine, flexible tubing. Once the patient is sedated, the biopsy capsule is placed at the back of the tongue using a tongue depressor. The depressor is withdrawn, the chin is held up and the child swallows the capsule. The tubing is advanced until the capsule is in the stomach. The child is then placed on his or her right side and the capsule is further advanced. It should fall towards the pylorus. Metoclopramide or cisapride administered via the tubing may be used to speed the passage of the capsule through the pylorus. Once the capsule is positioned in the desired site in the small intestine, it is fired by suction of the tubing with a 20-mL syringe. Larger and better-quality biopsies are provided by this technique, but it is time-consuming, can fail to deliver a biopsy and involves exposure to radiation.
- **Endoscopic biopsy:** this is quicker and provides a macroscopic view of the upper gastrointestinal tract. Multiple biopsies can be obtained, although they tend to be smaller.

The two techniques can be combined, by muzzle-loading a capsule into an endoscope, an approach which some consider to be the best compromise.

INDICATIONS

A biopsy of the small intestine is the investigation of choice when an enteropathy is suspected. The commonest enteropathies in children in general practice are coeliac disease, post-viral enteritis, cow's milk protein intolerance and giardiasis.

POTENTIAL FINDINGS

- Complete or partial villous atrophy may suggest coeliac disease, but not all children with an abnormal intestinal biopsy will have coeliac disease. Diseases such as post-viral enteritis may produce abnormalities which can be confused with coeliac disease and lead to inappropriate treatment. An experienced histopathologist is required to interpret the biopsy.

- Other diseases, such as cow's milk protein intolerance, may produce patchy non-specific changes.

RELATED INVESTIGATIONS

Small-bowel biopsy forms part of a structured approach to the investigation of children thought to have small-intestinal disease. The approach includes history, examination, assessment of growth, blood and stool investigations, barium studies and response to elimination diet (e.g. gluten, milk). Serum IgA class endomysial antibodies have a high specificity for coeliac disease, facilitating case-finding by GPs. Despite the availability of such screening tests, small-intestinal biopsy remains essential to the diagnosis.

PATIENT ADVICE

- Children need to fast for 6–8 hours, and babies for 4–6 hours.

- The child is sedated intravenously or orally.

- Patients should remain nil by mouth until the sedation has worn off (usually after 1–2 hours), but normally this is a day-case procedure.

- A doctor should be contacted if severe abdominal pain occurs or rectal bleeding is observed.

GP ADVICE

- Small-bowel biopsy is a safe procedure.
- The most serious complication is bleeding.
- Other complications include abdominal pain, bacteraemia and aspiration during passage of the tube or capsule.
- In one study series, no significant morbidity occurred after 3000 small-bowel biopsies.

RENAL MEDICINE

Urinary microscopy

Measurement of urinary protein excretion

Creatinine clearance

Renal ultrasound

Intravenous urogram (IVU)

Isotope renal scans (DTPA and DMSA)

Renal biopsy

CT scanning

Magnetic resonance imaging (MRI)

Magnetic resonance angiography (MRA)

Renal arteriography

RENAL MEDICINE

Mark Temple

The history and clinical examination form the basis for planning investigation in patients with suspected renal disease. In renal medicine, dipstick urinalysis is integral to the clinical examination and provides rapid additional information which helps to guide investigation.

Urinalysis is also routine in medical screening of healthy individuals in GP surgeries. Consequently, protocols are required for the appropriate investigation of asymptomatic patients with proteinuria or haematuria detected on dipstick testing.

Investigations in renal medicine address several principal questions.

- Is renal disease present?
- Is renal function impaired?
- Is the renal disease acute or chronic?
- What is the renal diagnosis?

Urinary microscopy

DESCRIPTION

A 10-mL sample of fresh midstream urine (MSU) is centrifuged at approximately 1500 rpm for 3 minutes. The supernatant is discarded and the sediment resuspended in 0.5 mL of urine. One drop of this suspension is examined by phase-contrast light microscopy.

INDICATIONS

- This is a simple, inexpensive assessment of any patient with abnormal dipstick urinalysis, with considerable potential to reduce unnecessary investigation.
- It is also used to confirm microscopic haematuria.

POTENTIAL FINDINGS

- Two or more red cells per high-power field confirms microscopic haematuria.
- Isolated haematuria is haematuria confirmed on microscopy in the absence of other features of renal disease (e.g. renal impairment or proteinuria).
- Red-cell casts (tubular structures consisting of red cells and a protein matrix) or dysmorphic red cells indicate glomerular disease (particularly if heavy proteinuria is present).
- Leucocyte casts are seen in acute bacterial pyelonephritis.

RELATED INVESTIGATIONS

- A MSU sample should be sent for urine culture, as urinary tract infection is a common cause of transient microscopic haematuria.
- Persistent haematuria requires further investigation. Renal tract malignancy is a particular cause for concern in older adults (e.g. > 40 years) without strong evidence of glomerular bleeding (proteinuria or red-cell casts), who should be referred to a urologist for cystoscopy.

Measurement of urinary protein excretion

DESCRIPTION

Twenty-four-hour urine collection is the gold standard for the quantification of proteinuria. All urine voided over a period of 24 hours is collected in a collecting bottle containing a small amount of preservative (e.g. thymol) obtained from the hospital clinical chemistry department.

A simple estimate of the 24-hour urine protein can be made from a single 'spot' urine specimen by measurement of the protein:creatinine ratio, which corrects for the degree of dilution of the urine.

Microalbuminuria (albumin excretion of 30–300 mg/day) is not detected on standard dipstick testing. Albumin is measured by a sensitive radioimmunoassay and expressed as the albumin:creatinine ratio from a spot urine specimen or as an albumin excretion rate on a timed urine specimen.

INDICATIONS

- Proteinuria on a single urine dipstick test is common. Transient proteinuria occurs in 4% of men and 7% of women, and does not require further investigation. Patients with persistent proteinuria (present on at least three occasions by dipstick testing) require further investigation.

- Quantifying the protein loss guides further investigation and may provide some prognostic information.

- Detection of microalbuminuria in diabetics suggests early diabetic nephropathy.

POTENTIAL FINDINGS

- Nephrotic-range proteinuria is the term given to heavy proteinuria (> 3.5 g/ 24 hours). Nephrotic syndrome consists of proteinuria > 3.5 g/24 hours, hypoalbuminaemia (serum albumin < 30 g/dL) and oedema.

- Isolated proteinuria is pathological proteinuria (> 300 mg/24 hours) in the absence of other features of renal disease (e.g. renal impairment).

- Microalbuminuria (albumin excretion of 30–300 mg/24 hours) is an important indicator of early diabetic nephropathy.

RELATED INVESTIGATIONS

- Increased proteinuria in the upright position (orthostatic proteinuria) is a benign condition that occurs in up to 5% of adolescents but is rare in adults over the age of 30 years. Urinalysis of early-morning urine (following recumbency) will be normal.

- Indications for a renal biopsy include nephrotic syndrome or less severe proteinuria associated with other signs of renal disease. Renal biopsy in patients with isolated proteinuria is generally recommended with proteinuria > 1 g/24 hours, as these patients are likely to have significant primary glomerular disease.

PATIENT ADVICE

- Twenty-four-hour urine collections are often incomplete. The patient should be advised to collect urine during a 24-hour period when they are likely to be at home.

- On waking, the patient should void normally into the toilet and thereafter collect all urine for the next 24 hours, completing the collection with the first urine voided on rising the following day.

- Placing the collection bottle in a prominent position or putting a note on the toilet door helps to remind the patient to collect all urine voided.

- The 24-hour urine collection should be returned to the hospital laboratory on the day of completion.

Creatinine clearance

DESCRIPTION

The glomerular filtration rate (GFR) is the best overall index of renal function. Accurate measurement of the GFR requires measurement of the clearance from the blood of a substance that is freely filtered in the glomerulus and neither secreted nor reabsorbed in the nephron.

The endogenous production of creatinine by muscle is relatively constant and easily measured, and creatinine is freely filtered by the glomerulus. Creatinine clearance is widely used to estimate the GFR.

Creatinine clearance is calculated from the total creatinine excreted in the urine over a timed period (e.g. 24 hours) and the serum creatinine measurement taken during the collection period.

INDICATIONS

- This is a more accurate estimate of renal function than serum creatinine or urea, which may be used to follow the progress of a disease or the patient's response to treatment.

- It is useful in patients for whom renal function assessed by serum creatinine is unreliable: low muscle mass – serum creatinine underestimates renal impairment (e.g. in the elderly, malnourished); increased muscle mass – raised serum creatinine reflects creatinine generation rather than renal impairment (e.g. muscular young adult males).

POTENTIAL FINDINGS

- Although creatinine is freely filtered by the glomerulus, it is also secreted by the tubules, and the creatinine clearance will overestimate GFR by 10–20% when renal function is near normal, and by a considerably greater amount when renal function is severely impaired.

- Incomplete urine collection will tend to result in an underestimate of renal function.

RELATED INVESTIGATIONS

- Inulin clearance accurately measures GFR as this substance is unaltered by the tubules. Inulin clearance is only used as a research tool.
- GFR can be calculated from the rate of disappearance of chromium-labelled EDTA (^{51}Cr-EDTA) from the blood. This method has the advantage of not requiring urine collection.

Renal ultrasound

DESCRIPTION

This is a widely used form of renal imaging which is quick and non-invasive.

INDICATIONS

It is commonly used early in the investigation of renal disease, as it may provide considerable diagnostic information (see below) (*see also* Urology chapter).

POTENTIAL FINDINGS

- Renal size and shape.
- Renal scarring (e.g. chronic pyelonephritis).
- Small kidneys (less than 8 cm in bipolar length) – suggests chronic renal disease.
- Single kidney – suggests previous nephrectomy or renal aplasia.
- Asymmetrical kidneys (bipolar length differs by >1 cm) – suggests renovascular disease.
- Renal parenchyma – cysts, tumours and polycystic kidney disease.
- Dilated renal pelvis and ureters – suggests obstructive nephropathy.
- Large post-micturition residual volume – suggests bladder outflow obstruction.
- Bladder mass – suggests tumour.
- Detection of renal stones (opaque and non-opaque).

RELATED INVESTIGATIONS

- Plain X-ray of the kidneys, ureter and bladder (KUB) is the best way of detecting calcification within the renal tract (most renal calculi are radio-opaque).
- An intravenous urogram (IVU) is often required to confirm whether calcification seen on KUB X-ray lies in the renal tract.
- Doppler ultrasound can be used to detect the abnormal renal artery waveform seen in renal artery stenosis.
- CT scanning for further assessment of renal masses.

PATIENT ADVICE

- Gel is applied to the skin on the abdomen with the patient recumbent and the ultrasound probe passed over the renal areas.
- A full bladder aids definition of bladder anatomy.
- Patients who require bladder imaging are advised to drink 1 pint of water 60–90 minutes before the scan and not to void urine until after the examination.

Intravenous urogram

DESCRIPTION

A series of X-rays is taken before and at timed intervals after intravenous injection of approximately 75 mL of contrast. The pre-contrast film is a KUB and, following intravenous injection, contrast is demonstrated in the renal parenchyma (nephrogram), collecting system (urogram), ureters and bladder.

INDICATIONS

- IVU has been largely superseded by renal ultrasound.
- It shows the detailed anatomy of the pelvicalyceal system and ureter.
- It is useful for accurate localisation of renal calculi.

POTENTIAL FINDINGS

- A 1-minute film taken immediately after the end of contrast injection serves as a measure of renal perfusion and provides information on renal size and shape.

- Later films provide images of the calyces and collecting system.

- A slowly developing, delayed nephrogram is characteristic of renal obstruction.

- In severe renal failure, contrast is not filtered by the glomeruli and no useful images are obtained.

RELATED INVESTIGATIONS

- See section on ultrasound.

- Antegrade and retrograde pyelography provide further information on ureteric obstruction and pathology of the renal pelvis and ureter. In obstructive uropathy, a nephrostomy catheter placed percutaneously in the renal pelvis is used to inject contrast (antegrade). In retrograde pyleography, contrast is injected into the lower ureter during cystoscopy.

PATIENT ADVICE

- The patient should provide details of any history of severe allergic reactions, particularly to iodine or radiographic contrast, as an IVU may be contra-indicated.

- In general, patients are advised to restrict their fluid intake to 500 mL during the 4 hours before the investigation, as the quality of the IVU is reduced in patients with dilute urine.

- To reduce the potential hazards of vomiting, the patient is asked not to eat for several hours before the IVU.

GP ADVICE

- A previous reaction to radiographic contrast increases the probability of a subsequent reaction by eightfold and a history of asthma increases it by sixfold. Alternative imaging should be considered in patients with a history of asthma or a serious reaction to radiographic contrast.

- Although contrast nephropathy is rare with the new, non-ionic radiographic agents, patients with diabetes or myeloma are at increased risk of this complication. If IVU is unavoidable, these patients should not be dehydrated prior to imaging.

Isotope renal scans (DTPA and DMSA)

1 DTPA scan – dynamic isotope renogram

DESCRIPTION

Dynamic imaging is provided by the isotope technetium-99m (99Tc) chelated to diethylenetriamine penta-acetic acid (DTPA) which, after intravenous injection, is filtered by the glomerulus. The DTPA isotope renogram has three phases, namely an initial vascular phase, a nephrogram and a final excretory phase. Excretion of the isotope in patients with dilated collecting systems may be slow, and this is due to pooling rather than to true obstruction. A brisk wash-out effect following administration of intravenous frusemide indicates pooling rather than obstruction.

INDICATIONS

- Assessment of renal arterial disease.
- Assessment of renal collecting system obstruction/dilation.

POTENTIAL FINDINGS

- Morphological information is inferior to that obtained by renal ultrasound or IVU.
- It provides functional information on renal blood flow and GFR.
- Renal artery stenosis is characterised by prolonged isotope uptake with a delayed second-phase peak.

RELATED INVESTIGATIONS

- See sections on IVU and ultrasound.
- A captopril renogram is used to screen for renal artery stenosis, and consists of a DTPA scan before and after a single dose of captopril. In renal artery stenosis, uptake of the isotope is reduced after captopril, due to an abrupt fall in post-glomerular arteriolar tone and reduced filtration pressure.
- CT and MRI are now more commonly used to screen for renovascular disease.

PATIENT ADVICE

- Scanning commences immediately after intravenous injection of approximately 0.5 mL of the medical isotope given as a bolus.

- The scan sequence takes about 1 hour to complete.

2 DMSA scan – static isotope renography

DESCRIPTION

Static imaging is provided by 99Tc dimercaptosuccinic acid (DMSA), which binds to the renal tubules, accurately reflecting the intrarenal distribution of functioning renal tissue.

INDICATIONS

- Assessment of renal parenchyma (e.g. scars – chronic pyelonephritis, infarcts).

- Assessment of divided renal function. The DMSA scan is a simple and reliable method of assessing the individual contribution of each kidney to total renal function (e.g. renal dysplasia, planning surgical intervention).

- Assessment of localisation of ectopic kidney.

POTENTIAL FINDINGS

- Demonstration of cortical scars (chronic pyelonephritis) is superior to that obtained with ultrasound.

- Cysts and tumours are not reliably distinguished, as both may have areas of non-functioning renal tissue.

- See above section on indications.

RELATED INVESTIGATIONS

See sections on ultrasound and IVU.

PATIENT ADVICE

- There is an interval of 4 hours between the intravenous injection of isotope and the commencement of scanning.

- The scanning takes about 30 minutes to complete.

Renal biopsy

DESCRIPTION

The patient lies prone for the biopsy procedure, and the lateral border of the lower pole of the kidney is located by ultrasound. The tissues are infiltrated with local anaesthetic and a Tru-Cut-type needle is either used manually or attached to a spring-loaded biopsy 'gun' in order to obtain renal tissue. Tissue is obtained for light and electron microscopy and immunofluorescence.

INDICATIONS

- Unexplained acute renal failure.
- Unexplained chronic renal failure (in cases where the kidneys are not small).
- Nephrotic syndrome (in adults).
- Persistent isolated proteinuria > 1 g/24 hours.
- Persistent microscopic haematuria (renal tract neoplasm excluded).
- Impaired renal transplant function.

Prompt renal biopsy is particularly important in cases where acute renal failure is unexplained, as the histology may reveal rapidly progressive glomerulonephritis that is amenable to immunosuppressive treatment. Biopsy should be avoided in patients with small, shrunken kidneys, obstructive nephropathy, reflux nephro-pathy or adult polycystic kidney disease. Renal imaging (usually by ultrasound) is performed before renal biopsy is arranged, to confirm the presence of two kidneys of normal size and shape. Small, shrunken kidneys (bipolar length < 8 cm) due to chronic renal failure are difficult to locate and biopsy safely, and renal histology is unlikely to be helpful. The presence of a single native kidney is often considered to be a contraindication to percutaneous renal biopsy, although histology can be obtained by an open surgical technique.

POTENTIAL FINDINGS

The appearance of renal tissue examined by light microscopy (augmented, where appropriate, by electron microscopy and immunofluorescence) allows histo-logical diagnosis of a wide range of renal disease, including glomerulonephritis, interstitial nephritis and vasculitis.

RELATED INVESTIGATIONS

Serum immunology may contribute to the diagnosis of certain forms of glomerulonephritis and vasculitis.

PATIENT ADVICE

- Hospital admission is required.
- Before the procedure, a venous blood sample is taken (for determinatin of full blood count and clotting status) and the patient's informed consent is obtained.
- The procedure is performed under local anaesthetic.
- Bruising at the site of renal puncture is common, but is rarely significant.
- The procedure takes about 45 minutes.
- Commonly, the patient remains recumbent in hospital for up to 24 hours after the biopsy, with regular monitoring of blood pressure and dipstick urinalysis.

GP ADVICE

- Haemorrhage is the most serious and common complication. A bleeding diathesis is an absolute contraindication to renal biopsy, and the patient's clotting status and platelet count must be checked prior to the procedure.
- Microscopic haematuria is common after the procedure, and macroscopic haematuria occurs in 5–10% of patients, with transfusion required in approximately 1% of cases.

CT scanning

Computerised tomography is valuable for detection of urinary tract pathology, and particularly for the assessment of renal and bladder tumours and peri-renal lesions. Rapid sequential imaging during the injection of intravenous contrast will provide information on renal artery patency. This information can be augmented by the recently developed technique of spiral CT scanning. The renal arteries are demonstrated accurately by coaxial CT scanning and manipulation of the images, allowing computerised reconstruction of anatomy in three dimensions.

Magnetic resonance imaging and magnetic resonance angiography

MRI provides similar information to that offered by CT scanning, but has the advantage that imaging can be obtained in any plane. Intravenous injection of a paramagnetic contrast medium, gadolinium DTPA, has allowed the development of MRA which, like spiral CT, has the ability to provide – non-invasively – sophisticated renal artery imaging.

Renal arteriography

Renal arteriography remains the gold standard for the demonstration of renal arterial anatomy. However, the technique is invasive, requiring injection of contrast into the aorta or directly into the renal arteries. Increasing numbers of patients with renovascular disease are being investigated and considered for renal artery angioplasty and stenting. These procedures require cannulation of the renal arteries and arteriography. Potential complications include arterial dissection and cholesterol embolisation. Digital subtraction angiography allows useful imaging of the renal arteries following the injection of an intravenous bolus of contrast. Images are manipulated digitally to optimise the angiography, although the images are inferior to those obtained by renal arteriography.

RESPIRATORY MEDICINE

Pulmonary function tests (PFTs)

Bronchoscopy

Lung biopsy

Radionuclide scanning

CT scanning

RESPIRATORY MEDICINE

Robert Stirling and Peter Barnes

Pulmonary function tests (PFTs)

DESCRIPTION AND INDICATIONS

- Appropriate PFTs are the key diagnostic tool in respiratory medicine. These tests may frequently prove diagnostic in themselves or when coupled with radiographic findings. At their simplest, PFTs involve forced breath manoeuvres into a spirometer that measures lung volume – forced expiratory volume in 1 second (FEV_1) and forced vital capacity (FVC). This detects the presence of airway obstruction or reduced lung volume, and may be performed on a regular basis in the GP surgery. More sophisticated volume measurements provide details of small airway function, gas trapping and hyperinflation. These tests require plethysmography, which is only available in a Lung Function Laboratory. Tests that measure inspiratory flow may be useful for diagnosing tracheal obstruction.

- Gas dilution techniques measure the ability of the alveoli to perform their principal task, namely that of gas transfer, using the tracer gas carbon monoxide (CO).

- Lung-volume testing can be allied to non-specific or specific challenge testing to demonstrate airway hyper-reactivity. Histamine (or methacholine) challenge defines airway hyper-reactivity as the challenge concentration required to cause a defined fall in FEV_1 – typically a 20% fall in FEV_1 reported as PC_{20}. Additional challenges may be useful when clinical findings suggest specific reactivity (e.g. in exercise-induced, cold-induced or occupational asthma), although these results should generally be interpreted in consultation with a specialist.

- Tests that measure respiratory muscle strength are indicated in patients who have neuromuscular-skeletal disorders and respiratory symptoms.

- Arterial blood gases (PaO_2, $PaCO_2$) are measured in patients with severe obstructive lung diseases when long-term oxygen therapy is under consideration.

- PFTs are invaluable in tailoring treatment to disease. In chronic obstructive pulmonary disease (COPD), repeated spirometry can be used to identify steroid responsiveness and treatment benefits in response to inhalers and nebulisers. Bronchodilator responsiveness can also be measured.

POTENTIAL FINDINGS

- PFTs provide the diagnoses and measures of disease severity necessary for treatment and definition of the prognosis.

- Spirometry and gas-transfer results will be reported both as absolute values and as a percentage of 'normal'. In general, values of $\geqslant$ 80% of predicted normal fall within normal limits, values of 50–80% represent a mild to moderate reduction and values of $\leqslant$ 50% indicate a severe reduction.

- Table 1 summarises some common findings.

Table 1

	FEV₁/FVC	*Gas transfer*	*Bronchodilator reversibility*
Normal	> 80%	> 80%	< 12–15%
Asthma	Ratio reduced; FVC normal/increased	Normal or increased	+
COPD: emphysema	Ratio reduced; FVC normal/increased	Reduced	–
chronic bronchitis	Ratio reduced; FVC normal/increased	Normal	+/–
Interstitial lung disease	Ratio normal or increased; FVC decreased	Preserved early; reduced late	–

RELATED INVESTIGATIONS

- **Fitness to fly:** by simulating air-cabin hypoxia, peripheral oxygen desaturation can be measured, enabling assessment of 'fitness to fly' in patients with the potential to develop hypoxia.

- **Exercise testing:** reduced oxygen extraction limits exercise tolerance. Exercise testing may therefore determine the pulmonary contribution to exercise limitation as opposed to limitations due to cardiac, musculo-skeletal and volitional factors. These tests must be performed in a specialist Lung Function Laboratory.

- **Echocardiography**: findings of right heart failure in COPD suggest cor pulmonale.

PATIENT ADVICE

- No preparation is necessary for these tests, although use of asthma 'relievers' (β-agonists) will need to be suspended prior to bronchodilator response and challenge tests.

- Some patients feel claustrophobic while using a nose clamp and when inside the plethysmograph ('body box'), but this is rarely a significant problem.

- Blood gas analysis involves either a small syringe or lancet sampling from the wrist (or, in some centres, the earlobe).

GP ADVICE

- Clinical details – giving detailed patient information on investigation requests helps the Lung Function Laboratory to streamline investigations.

- Infection control – laboratory spirometers involve extensive breathing circuits, which cannot always be completely changed between patients. Therefore any suspected or known active infection should be brought to the attention of laboratory staff so that precautions may be taken.

- Preparation – if challenge testing or bronchodilator responsiveness is requested, the patient should be instructed not to use either long- or short-acting β-agonists on the morning prior to testing.

- The following contraindications should be borne in mind:
    - (i)   active pulmonary infection (e.g. Pneumocystis pneumonia or TB (all tests));
    - (ii) previous severe asthma exacerbations (challenge tests);
    - (iii) comorbidity (e.g. ischaemic heart disease) (challenge tests).

Bronchoscopy

DESCRIPTION

Fibre-optic bronchoscopy (FOB) allows direct visualisation of both upper and lower respiratory tract as far as the fourth- or fifth-generation airways. This procedure is particularly effective for disease processes that affect the alveoli and lumen (e.g. infection, alveolar haemorrhage) or the airway wall (e.g. neoplasia, asthma, sarcoidosis), but is less effective for evaluation of pulmonary parenchymal diseases.

The use of fine forceps enables visually directed mucosal biopsy, although distal lung tissue/masses may be sampled blindly by trans-tracheal or trans-bronchial biopsy. Lumenal cells may be retrieved for analysis by lavage, while airway wall cells (mainly epithelium) can be retrieved using a fine 'bottlebrush'.

INDICATIONS

Evaluation of the following:

- haemoptysis;
- chronic cough;
- pulmonary nodule/infiltrate;
- acute/chronic infection;
- diagnosis and staging of lung cancer;
- monitoring lung-transplant grafts.

POTENTIAL FINDINGS

Few conditions have pathognomonic bronchoscopic findings (neoplasia, pulmonary alveolar proteinosis, pulmonary haemorrhage). Findings must therefore be examined within the clinical context.

PATIENT ADVICE

- The modern bronchoscope is a flexible, fine device with a video camera at its tip, which can be passed rapidly and safely via the nose or mouth into the lungs. The tube is sufficiently narrow (3–4 mm) for it not to affect air movement during normal breathing.

- Bronchoscopy frequently requires some light sedation, and it is therefore important that no food or liquid is taken for 8 hours prior to the procedure. Sedation is given via a small needle in a peripheral vein, usually in the form of a short-acting sedative-hypnotic or anaesthetic.

- The throat and nasal passages are anaesthetised using a topical spray. This anaesthesia may predispose to aspiration, and the patient must not take food or liquid for 2 hours after the anaesthesia.

- The procedure generally takes 20–30 minutes, is slightly uncomfortable and may induce cough.
- Minor haemoptysis is common following procedures involving biopsy but usually clears within 6 hours.
- Following anaesthesia it is recommended that the patient is collected from the hospital by a friend or relative and does not drive.

GP ADVICE

- Clear clinical details must be provided for the bronchoscopist to ensure detailed, directed examination and so that all appropriate investigations are carried out.
- Patients and radiography are generally evaluated within a specialist unit prior to bronchoscopy and the results made available either through the clinic or the GP surgery.
- Full blood count and coagulation results must be available prior to procedures in which brush or biopsy forceps are used.
- Contraindications include coagulopathy and pulmonary hypertension.

Lung biopsy

DESCRIPTION

- Lung biopsy is now performed by video-assisted thoracoscopic surgery (VATS), a minimally invasive surgical technique which is available in most surgical centres.
- VATS provides satisfactory exposure and sampling opportunities but reduces incisional size, post-operative discomfort and the duration of in-patient stay required.

INDICATIONS

If a diagnosis cannot be achieved by less invasive procedures, and if diagnostic inclusion or exclusion will positively influence outcome, then lung biopsy may be indicated in the following situations:

- lung mass;

- persistent chest X-ray infiltrate;
- interstitial lung disease;
- atypical infection.

POTENTIAL FINDINGS

- Neoplasia – primary lung carcinoma, secondary lung tumour.
- Fibrosing alveolitis/scarring.
- Infection.
- Non-neoplastic infiltrative disease (e.g. vasculitis, eosinophilic pneumonia, amyloid).

PATIENT ADVICE

- Lung biopsy involves surgical removal of a small amount of lung tissue for detailed pathological and microbiological examination.
- The procedure may now be performed using a keyhole technique, which markedly reduces pain, wound size and the duration of hospitalisation needed.
- The patient will have a general anaesthetic and a tube will be passed into the lung to assist the patient's breathing while he or she is asleep.
- The patient normally has to stay in hospital for 2–3 days after the operation.
- The operation wound generally heals quickly, but less commonly it may remain sore for several weeks. This discomfort can normally be controlled by simple over-the-counter painkillers. Rarely, the lung may fail to inflate properly after the operation, but this can be managed simply with a chest drain.

GP ADVICE

Lung biopsy is an invasive operative procedure and should only be performed after communication between GP, physician and thoracic surgeon. A clear understanding of the influence of potential results on management outcomes is needed before proceeding with the biopsy.

Radionuclide scanning

- Radionuclide scanning of the lungs is of particular importance in determining patterns of ventilation and match or mismatch with pulmonary perfusion. This is a key diagnostic test in pulmonary embolism, but it is also useful for identifying under-ventilated lung segments prior to surgery such as lobectomy, transplantation or lung-volume reduction.

- These scans involve the inhalation of taste-free radiolabels (krypton, xenon or technetium) and subsequent scanning of their deposition within the lung fields using a gamma camera.

- Pulmonary epithelial integrity in interstitial lung disease may be assessed using DTPA scanning, providing important prognostic information.

- There are no strict contraindications to these nuclear investigations but, as always, it is preferable to avoid them during pregnancy.

CT scanning

- CT scanning provides high-resolution investigation of chest structures using a variation of the standard X-ray. High-resolution imaging is achieved by taking thin-section images, allowing better assessment of the parenchyma. Single CT scans deliver 50–100 times the radiation dose of a single chest X-ray, but are still considered to be quite safe.

- CT scanning is invaluable for assessing the mediastinum, pleura and lung parenchyma, and in combination with contrast material it delineates major vascular structures.

- Iodinated contrast is most widely used for radiological studies. These dyes are introduced intravenously and may provide a warm, flushing sensation that lasts for a few seconds. Renal impairment, diabetes and asthma are all relative contraindications to contrast material, and the operator needs to be aware of these comorbidities.

UROLOGY

Uroflowmetry

Urodynamic studies

Ultrasound

Scrotal ultrasound

Flexible cystoscopy

Transrectal ultrasound and biopsy of the prostate

Urine cytology

UROLOGY

Ciaran Brady

Uroflowmetry

DESCRIPTION

In many units, this test is performed in the radiology department. The patient, either standing or sitting, is asked to void into a device that measures the volume of urine voided per unit time (mL/second). This results in a bell-shaped curve in the normal subject.

INDICATIONS

- Uroflowmetry is indicated as part of the assessment of voiding disorders in combination with urological history, examination and a frequency–volume chart.
- Uroflowmetry is now standard practice in the selection of patients for prostate surgery whose lower urinary tract symptoms are suggestive of benign prostatic obstruction.

POTENTIAL FINDINGS

- Normal uroflow and complete emptying – however, this does not exclude early benign prostatic obstruction or detrusor instability.
- Low flow rate and complete emptying, suggesting outflow obstruction and/or detrusor failure.
- High flow rate and complete emptying, suggesting abdominal straining in the normal subject or detrusor instability without obstruction.
- Low flow rate and incomplete emptying, suggesting outflow obstruction and detrusor failure.
- Intermittent flow rate and variable emptying, suggesting detrusor failure and abdominal straining.

RELATED INVESTIGATIONS

- Uroflowmetry is often combined with ultrasound scanning before and after uroflowmetry to assess the upper tracts, bladder-wall morphology and post-micturition residual urine.
- Women mostly complain of symptoms that are related to storage rather than voiding, and are therefore investigated primarily with urodynamic studies.

PATIENT ADVICE

The patient should attend with a comfortably full bladder and void normally (an overfull bladder will not contract as strongly or empty as efficiently).

GP ADVICE

The maximum flow rate (Q_{max}) and the mean flow rate (Q_{ave}) are calculated electronically and can be misleading – the uroflow curve must also be assessed in conjunction for interpretation. Similarly, the time to Q_{max} and voiding time may not be representative of the patient's routine voiding pattern. It is preferable for the patient to attend a 'flow clinic' and take part in several uroflow studies, as a single study may underestimate the Q_{max}, and the patient may be influenced by inhibitory factors during the first study.

Urodynamic studies (UDS)

DESCRIPTION

UDS consist of cystometry and urethral pressure profilometry (UPP). They investigate the cause of the patient's symptoms by correlating them with objective measurements of physiological parameters. UDS are invasive and involve passing a filling catheter and a bladder-pressure line through the urethra and inserting another pressure line into the rectum. The bladder is emptied and then gently filled with warmed sodium chloride solution at slow, medium or fast filling rates. Information on bladder storage functions, namely sensation, capacity, detrusor compliance and stability, and urethral competency is provided in the filling phase. At regular intervals, urethral competency is assessed by Valsalva straining and coughing. Various tests may also be used to provoke unstable detrusor contractions. After filling, a voiding study is performed to assess urethral function and the pressure generated by the detrusor, which is correlated with uroflowmetry. In UPP, a catheter connected to a pressure transducer is withdrawn from the urethra at a fixed rate.

INDICATIONS

- UDS provide useful data on all of the parameters outlined above.
- They are particularly useful for the assessment of mixed incontinence and in demonstrating different types of stress incontinence, thereby influencing the subsequent surgical approach.
- The voiding study may help to identify patients with detrusor failure who may not necessarily benefit from prostate surgery.
- Patients with clinically diagnosed bladder overactivity who have not responded to empirical treatment should also have UDS performed.

POTENTIAL FINDINGS

Filling phase:

- decreased compliance;
- decreased capacity;
- altered sensation;
- detrusor instability;
- sphincteric incompetence.

Voiding phase:

- prostate/bladder neck obstruction;
- detrusor failure;
- urethral stricture.

RELATED INVESTIGATIONS

- Video-urodynamics (this allows dynamic visualisation of the bladder and urethra).
- Uroflowmetry.
- Cystoscopy.

PATIENT ADVICE

- The patient is asked to empty his or her bladder before the study.
- UDS may take up to 45 minutes to perform.
- The urethral catheters are passed using local anaesthetic lubricant.
- Dysuria for up to 1 day is common, but if symptoms persist, medical advice should be sought, as infection can occur as a result of the test.

GP ADVICE

- Dysuria following this procedure is not uncommon and settles within 1–2 days; send a MSU and treat for UTI if symptoms persist.
- In the presence of an otherwise normal history, examination and urinalysis, UDS are not required in cases of bladder overactivity. These cases may be treated empirically.

Ultrasound

DESCRIPTION

This test can provide sufficient information for diagnosis of diverse urological pathologies in both the upper and lower urinary tracts and testes. Ultrasound examination is quick, non-invasive and does not involve radioactivity. For these reasons, it has replaced the IVU as the initial investigation of choice for most upper tract symptoms.

INDICATIONS

- Cases of haematuria, loin pain, renal failure, recurrent UTIs or lower urinary tract symptoms may all be investigated using ultrasound.
- In the bladder, post-micturition residual urine volume may be calculated. Although ultrasound can provide useful information about the morpohology of the bladder wall, it is no substitute for flexible cystoscopy.
- Scrotal ultrasound – see below.
- *See also* the renal medicine section.

For further information on potential findings, related investigations and patient advice, see the Renal medicine chapter.

Scrotal ultrasound

This is useful in the following situations.

- **Torsion**: the main differential diagnosis is epididymo-orchitis, and in the vast majority of cases where testicular torsion is suspected, colour Doppler ultrasound of the scrotum will confirm the diagnosis.
- **Trauma**: ultrasound will identify a fractured testis and distinguish between haematoma and herniated testicular tissue. Not infrequently, malignancies may underlie a scrotal swelling, which the patient attributes to 'trauma'.
- **Malignancy**: ultrasound assessment of the painless testicular mass will distinguish betwen intra- and extra-testicular masses; tumours have a characteristic appearance.
- **Varicoceles, epididymal cysts and hydroceles**: ultrasound is indicated in these conditions only when the presentation or physical findings are atypical.

Flexible cystoscopy

DESCRIPTION

This short procedure is generally tolerated extremely well using local anaesthetic lubricant. The flexible fibrescope is passed, giving a magnified, high-resolution image of the urethra, prostate and entire bladder. It is possible to take biopsies with minimal discomfort.

INDICATIONS

- Follow-up of patients with carcinoma of the bladder.
- Investigation of frank haematuria/microhaematuria.
- Investigation of recurrent UTIs.
- Investigation of lower urinary tract symptoms which are suggestive of benign prostatic obstruction but are either atypical or unresponsive to medical therapy.

POTENTIAL FINDINGS

- **Urethra:** stricture, urethritis, carcinoma, urethral valves/congenital anomalies.
- **Prostate:** elongation of gland, occlusive lobes, inflammation, tumour, post-operative bladder neck stricture.
- **Bladder:** residual urine, trabeculation/diverticulae, increased (or decreased) capacity, inflammation, carcinoma, stone.

RELATED INVESTIGATIONS

- Intravenous urography.
- Renal ultrasound.

PATIENT ADVICE

- The patient is asked to empty his or her bladder before the study.
- The procedure takes less than 5 minutes and is performed under local anaesthesia.
- Dysuria for up to 1 day is common, but if symptoms persist, the patient should be advised to seek medical attention, as UTIs can occur as a result of the test.
- If a biopsy is taken, intermittent, light bleeding may occur for 1–2 days.

GP ADVICE

Dysuria and haematuria following this procedure are not uncommon, and settle within 1–2 days. Send a MSU specimen and treat the patient for UTI if symptoms persist.

Transrectal ultrasound (TRUS) and biopsy of the prostate

DESCRIPTION

The patient lies in the left lateral position, and a digital rectal examination (DRE) of the prostate is performed. The ultrasound probe is then placed in the insensate lower rectum to assess the volume, shape and echotexture of the gland. Although

TRUS of the prostate alone is very sensitive to prostate cancer, biopsies are taken from the upper, middle and lower aspect of each lateral lobe to confirm the diagnosis ('sextant biopsies'). Biopsies provide histological information about grade, stage and the extension to the capsular margin and/or invasion of the seminal vesicles. Suspicious nodules are biopsied directly. In addition, seminal vesicle biopsies are often taken in patients who may be candidates for radical prostatectomy.

INDICATIONS

- Abnormal DRE and/or raised level of prostate-specific antigen (PSA).
- To confirm a suspected diagnosis of prostate cancer prior to commencing treatment.
- As a staging procedure to assist in the selection of patients for radical prostatectomy.

POTENTIAL FINDINGS

- Symmetrical enlargement is characteristic of a (benign) prostate adenoma.
- Hypoechoic signs and irregularity or discontinuity of the capsular echoes are characteristic of carcinoma of the prostate.
- Acute inflammatory changes are secondary to oedema and are characteristic. Findings in chronic prostatitis are varied, and they change as the condition evolves, making diagnosis difficult.
- Biopsies provide histological information as described above.

RELATED INVESTIGATIONS

- PSA testing.
- Cystoscopy.

PATIENT ADVICE

- The test takes about 10 minutes to perform.
- It is uncomfortable, and can be painful, but general anaesthesia is rarely required.
- As the test is performed transrectally, antibiotic prophylaxis is required to minimise the risk of sepsis. Different regimens are employed in each centre.

- Preparation of the bowel is not required.
- Haematuria can occur for 1 or 2 days after the test.

GP ADVICE

If symptoms of sepsis occur, the patient should be sent to hospital urgently.

Urine cytology

DESCRIPTION

Malignant transitional epithelial cells lose their adhesive properties and so are shed into the urine. Cells from high-grade tumours and carcinoma *in situ* are more likely to be shed, and therefore cytology has a poor sensitivity for detecting well-differentiated and moderately well-differentiated tumours. Overall, the sensitivity of cytology in detecting malignancy is 80%. However, when cytology is repeated several times in patients with a history of transitional-cell carcinoma (TCC), the sensitivity increases to > 95%.

INDICATIONS

- TCC presents in the majority of cases as painless haematuria. All patients with haematuria therefore require cytology, cystoscopy and upper tract imaging.
- 'Irritative' symptoms associated with malignancy very rarely occur in the absence of haematuria. However, prior to treating such cases, many urologists send a specimen for cytology.
- Surveillance for recurrence of TCC.

POTENTIAL FINDINGS

- Cells may be described as malignant, suspicious of malignancy or atypical.
- Inflammatory cells and bacteria may also be identified.
- Artefactual cytological changes occur with UTIs, catherisation, calculi and following instrumentation of the urinary tract.
- False-positive results may be caused by atypia, inflammation or previous intravesical chemotherapy or external-beam radiotherapy.

RELATED INVESTIGATIONS

- Cystoscopy.
- Urography/ultrasound.

PATIENT ADVICE

- Immediately after shedding, degradation of the cell occurs and therefore specimens should be very fresh – preferably provided at the hospital.
- First-voided morning specimens are unsuitable, as they contain many dead cells which have been shed overnight.

GP ADVICE

Most people who die from bladder cancer do so from distant metastases and have a past history of TCC. Regular cytology and cystoscopy will detect recurrent disease and increase survival.

VASCULAR SURGERY

Angiography

Doppler studies

Ultrasound for aneurysms

VASCULAR SURGERY

David Reilly

Management of vascular patients is undergoing rapid change, not only because of the availability of more non-invasive tests, but also because of the recognition that most patients will be managed non-operatively.

Vascular patients are very variably catered for around the country, and access to both specialist advice and further investigations depends on the local situation. In some areas, for example, GPs will have open access to vascular laboratory tests such as Doppler scanning, and in other areas an appointment at the vascular clinic will be required first.

In order to gain the maximum benefit from vascular tests, it is important to be selective. For example, there is no point in performing invasive tests such as an angiogram unless intervention is planned, and this can only be decided by the responsible specialist. Protocols for referral should be locally agreed between GPs and specialists.

Direct access to interventional vascular radiology has developed in some countries, but in the UK the safest approach has been found to be close co-operation between radiologist and surgeon, in order to decide in a rapidly changing field whether an open, endovascular or conservative approach is most appropriate.

This chapter looks at the vascular investigations which should be available as part of a local vascular service, either directly to the GP or via a specialist clinic.

Angiography

INDICATIONS

Angiography is not directly available to the GP but via a vascular referral. Angiography is generally synonymous with arteriography. The aim is to provide anatomical information about the arterial tree, i.e. a 'road-map' for planning intervention. Most vascular units now use computer-enhanced imaging, known as either digital subtraction angiography (DSA) or digital vascular imaging (DVI). This allows the use of smaller injection cannulae and lower volumes of contrast, so is safer than previous techniques and can often be performed as a day-case procedure in fitter, uncomplicated cases.

DESCRIPTION

There are a variety of routes, of which the following are the commonest.

- **Transfemoral aortogram:** the commonest approach to contrast studies of the aorta and its branches is via a puncture under local anaesthetic of the femoral artery in the groin. This will be used, for example, to assess suitability for percutaneous angioplasty, or to determine whether a planned bypass graft is feasible.

- **Translumbar aortogram:** this route is used if no femoral pulses are palpable. It usually requires general anaesthesia and has a 1% serious complication rate (e.g. internal bleeding).

- **Arch angiogram:** the transfemoral route is used to thread a catheter into the arch of the aorta to cannulate subclavian vessels for upper-arm ischaemia. This route is now seldom used to perform carotid angiography. Because of the 2% stroke risk, it has been largely replaced by colour Doppler scanning.

- **Brachial angiogram:** if imaging of arm vessels is required, the transfemoral route to the brachial artery is used. If lower-limb vessel imaging is required, but aorta or iliac vessels are occluded, the catheter can be inserted into the brachial artery in the antecubital fossa.

POTENTIAL FINDINGS

Sometimes, if a lesion such as a short stenosis or occlusion is found, the radiologist may proceed with balloon angioplasty. This will depend on discussion of the suitability of the procedure with the vascular surgeon. More commonly, because of time constraints or bed availability, this is scheduled for later, and the patient will be reviewed in the vascular clinic to decide whether surgery or angioplasty is technically feasible and appropriate.

RELATED INVESTIGATIONS

- **MRA:** this is developing rapidly and may increasingly replace the more invasive contrast angiography in the future. It cannot be used in patients who suffer from claustrophobia or have metallic implants.

- **Exercise testing:** the first diagnostic decision involving a vascular patient may concern whether peripheral vascular disease is present or not – the patient may give a history suggestive of intermittent claudication but have normal ankle pressure. Exercise testing can elucidate this. The principle is that if there is a moderate stenosis in the artery, the ankle pressure can be normal when the flow is low, but after exercise – such as a treadmill – the increased flow into the muscle will cause a pressure drop over the stenosis.

PATIENT ADVICE

The local radiology department should supply detailed information as to whether local or general anaesthesia is planned, and whether fasting or an overnight stay are required, as these factors are so variable.

GP ADVICE

The main problems and risks associated with angiography are contrast toxicity, allergy or overload, pain and discomfort for the patient (which may necessitate sedation), and occasional arterial occlusion (due to dissecting up a flap of intima) or distal embolisation. The risks are small but real, and this means that angiograms should be performed only in a unit with full medical and vascular surgical back-up.

Doppler studies

Doppler investigations range from the many uses of the simple hand-held Doppler to scanning using the colour ('duplex') Doppler. The simple device detects blood flow and direction by bouncing high-frequency sound off red cells. The characteristics of the signal also provide useful information. The much more expensive Doppler scanners require an experienced operator, and combine imaging of the artery with flow velocity, so provide functional information about the significance of any stenosis found.

1 Hand-held Doppler probes

INDICATIONS

To assess peripheral vascular disease. Hand-held Doppler probes are routinely used in vascular clinics and increasingly used in primary care.

POTENTIAL FINDINGS

An indication of the severity of vascular disease is given by the ratio of the pressure measured in an artery at the ankle to the systolic pressure in the brachial artery – the ankle brachial pressure index (ABPI). This index is of use to district nurses when applying graduated compression bandages, which should not be applied without vascular advice if the ABPI is < 0.8. The absolute pressure is also useful, as ischaemic rest pain or ulceration is unlikely to improve spontaneously below a pressure of 50 mmHg.

PATIENT ADVICE

A sphygmomanometer cuff is placed above the ankle, the vessel with the clearest signal (usually the posterior tibial or dorsalis pedis) is located and the cuff is inflated until the signal disappears. The cuff is then gradually deflated until the signal reappears and that pressure is recorded.

2 Colour Doppler scans

(a) Carotid Doppler scan

DESCRIPTION

An ultrasound probe is placed over the area of interest and the vessel is identified.

INDICATIONS

For patients with TIAs in whom carotid surgery is being considered.

POTENTIAL FINDINGS

Depending on operator experience, a highly accurate estimation of the degree of carotid stenosis can be made, sufficient to enable a decision to be made about proceeding to carotid endarterectomy. This has now largely replaced carotid angiography.

RELATED INVESTIGATIONS

If the artery is heavily calcified or the stenosis is very tight, it may be difficult to be sure of patency or the degree of stenosis. In this case, an MRA scan may be recommended.

PATIENT ADVICE

- It usually takes about 20–30 minutes to test both carotids.
- The procedure is risk-free, painless and is performed with the patient reclining on a couch.

(b) Venous scanning

DESCRIPTION

The whole length of the leg is assessed with the ultrasound probe, identifying veins and determining whether or not blood flow is present. In experienced hands, the colour Doppler can replace the need for invasive venography.

INDICATIONS

Suspected deep vein thrombosis (DVT) (clinical diagnosis of DVT is very inaccurate).

POTENTIAL FINDINGS

Patients with negative scans, and those with calf-vein thrombosis extending no further than the popliteal vein, can avoid admission. The latter condition can be treated at home with mobilisation and anticoagulation. More extensive thrombosis may require in-patient management, depending on local practice.

RELATED INVESTIGATIONS

- **Venography:** this requires cannulation of a foot vein (which can be difficult to find), the injection of irritant contrast material and the application of a tourniquet. It can be painful and time-consuming, but until recently has been regarded as the most accurate test for DVT. It is now being replaced by non-invasive duplex Doppler scanning.
- Various other tests that attempt to filter out patients with a low likelihood of DVT are in use. These are inaccurate, but if entirely normal they do exclude a DVT. If abnormal results are obtained, a formal investigation such as Doppler scanning or venography is recommended. Such tests include thermography (in which a thermal photographic print of the leg is taken) and compression ultrasound.

PATIENT ADVICE

If colour Doppler scanning is available, it is accurate and pain- and risk-free. Venography is accurate, but will require an injection in the foot, can be painful, and usually requires admission.

GP ADVICE

Local availability and protocols will determine which tests can be used, but both colour Doppler scanning and venography are reliable.

Ultrasound for aneurysms

DESCRIPTION

Ultrasound scanning for the presence or absence of an aortic aneurysm is quick, accurate and often performed by an ultrasonographer with a mobile screening unit.

INDICATIONS

- Clinical suspicion of aortic aneurysm.
- A strong case can also be made for aneurysm screening, which is now available in several areas of the country. However, health authorities will not fund population screening until the final results of national studies are reported.

POTENTIAL FINDINGS

The most reproducible measurement is the maximum antero-posterior diameter, and it is this that interests the vascular surgeon. If an aortic aneurysm (defined as 3 cm in diameter or over) is found, then yearly scans are recommended. If the aorta is 5 cm in diameter or over, or is increasing in size by 1 cm per year, vascular referral is recommended unless this is contraindicated by extreme age or frailty.

RELATED INVESTIGATIONS

If it is unclear from the ultrasound scan whether the aneurysm extends above the renal arteries, then a CT scan will be recommended, as suprarenal surgery is considerably more hazardous and may require tertiary referral.

PATIENT ADVICE

The scan is painless, takes about 5 minutes and needs no special preparation.

GP ADVICE

Opportunistic screening is relatively cheap, and is particularly indicated in men over 60 years of age with peripheral vascular disease or hypertension, or other risk factors such as familial hyperlipidaemia or a first-degree relative with an aneurysm.

Index